Bioavailability of Drugs

Proceedings of the Conference on Bioavailability of Drugs at the National Academy of Sciences of the United States, Washington, D.C., November 22–23, 1971

Bioavailability of Drugs

Editors:

B.B. Brodie
Consultant, National Heart and Lung Institute, National Institutes of Health, Bethesda, Md.

W.M. Heller
Executive Director, United States Pharmacopeial Convention, Inc., Rockville, Md.

87 figures and 18 tables

S. Karger · Basel · München · Paris · London · New York · Sydney · 1972

Reprint from 'Pharmacology', Vol. 8, No. 1–3, 1972

S. Karger · Basel · München · Paris · London · New York · Sydney
Arnold-Böcklin-Strasse 25, CH–4011 Basel (Switzerland)

Printed in Switzerland by Thür Offsetdruck, Birsfelden
ISBN 3–8055–1456–5

Contents

Conference Data

Publication of the Proceedings is through an enabling grant provided by the Pharmaceutical Manufacturers Association.

Support for the Conference was through enabling grants provided by the Food and Drug Administration and the Pharmaceutical Manufacturers Association Foundation, Inc.

Sponsors of the Conference

- Academy of Pharmaceutical Sciences of the American Pharmaceutical Association
- Drug Research Board of the National Academy of Sciences–National Research Council
- Food and Drug Administration
- National Formulary
- Pharmaceutical Manufacturers Association Foundation, Inc.
- United States Pharmacopeia

Preface

The bioavailability of a drug substance in man relates to its appearance in the general circulation following administration in a pharmaceutical dosage form. The controversial question of drug product equivalence is allied to potential variations in bioavailability depending upon the properties of different drug formulations and other complex factors.

In the interest of the patient, the practitioner seeks confidence that the medication he prescribes or dispenses will possess optimal bioavailability, and turns to the standards and regulating agencies for such reassurance. As a result, there is no other, single, more important problem facing the compendia today than to work toward the development of uniform standards of performance in this important area of drug quality.

The purpose of this Conference on the Bioavailability of Drugs, therefore, is to bring together knowledgeable scientists from the pharmaceutical industry, government, universities, and other institutions, as well as practitioners, in order to assess the current status and to assist the compendia in their difficult task.

Welcome Addresses

This is not just another conference on bioavailability. This is not a conference to report new and interesting data, although some of our speakers may do that, too. This *is* a conference to open up the consideration of official, public standards of bioavailability, to be met by all sizes, strengths and brands of a United States Pharmacopeia (USP) drug product.

The Food and Drug Law empowers the Food and Drug Administration (FDA) to enforce the standards of strength, quality, purity, packaging and labeling of drug products included in the USP and the National Formulary. The scientists (researchers and educators) and the practitioners (physicians and pharmacists) of America have a unique privilege. Ours is the only country in the world where the people grant to the professions the privilege of writing the standards of quality for the drug products they will use. In America, the standards are not established by the drug producers nor the regulators, but by the professions that must know and appreciate the standards in order to select and use drug products wisely on behalf of the patient.

For the USP, the standards are the province of the Committee of Revision. These men are volunteers elected by their peers in a nationwide system involving all the schools of medicine and pharmacy and the state and national associations of both professions, as well as certain national organizations such as the Pharmaceutical Manufacturers Association (PMA) and certain federal agencies such as the FDA.

It is especially appropriate that this biprofessional body is responsible for establishing public standards of *bioavailability,* for this is surely the area where the supporting sciences of both professions merge most intimately. The USP Subcommittee on Bioavailability is composed almost equally of clinical pharmacologists from medicine and biopharmaceutical specialists from pharmacy. And because USP *also* represents practitioners, we can expect any standards to be chosen because they are useful and needed in the best practice of the two professions, not just because the current state of science permits us to answer an interesting question. After all, the production of drugs in this country is already more reliable than other aspects of the medication system, such as maintenance of quality through the various steps of dose preparation and administration at the practitioner and patient level. To add additional tests at the manufacturing level that would not help the practitioner or the patient utilize the drugs more advantageously, would do little for the patient except increase his drug bill.

When USP asked the Drug Research Board to co-sponsor this conference with us, it was our purpose to put on a conference that would permit an exposure of the views of a broad segment of the health community. Obviously, the overwhelming attendance attests to the vital interest in this subject. It also precludes more than a brief *exchange* of views. We would urge you, then, to continue to follow USP progress in this area and to let us know of your concerns and of information you have that might be useful to the Subcommittee on Bioavailability. Although chairman *Azarnoff* is from just across the line in Kansas, I think the USP Subcommittee on Bioavailability might adopt two mottoes from Missouri for the next couple of years: (1) the buck stops here, and (2) show me.

Ladies and gentlemen, distinguished speakers, representatives of our co-sponsoring organizations, hardworking staff members of the host organizations, it is my pleasure to bid you welcome on behalf of the Board of Trustees and the Committee of Revision of The United States Pharmacopeia.

May this conference be a milestone in the long road toward optimal drug therapy.

William M. Heller, Ph.D.
Executive Director, The United States Pharmacopeial Convention, Inc.

On behalf of the PMA, I wish to welcome all of you to this conference on a matter of substantial interest to the pharmaceutical industry. Many times over the last five years the pharmaceutical industry, through the Foundation, has sponsored and supported a number of meetings which we have judged to provide the occasion for a responsible discussion of an important matter, as we so judged this meeting.

With the Drug Research Board, we have supported workshops and conferences on drug metabolism, immunopharmacology, clinical investigations, clinical pharmacology, adverse reactions, and mutagenicity. The interest in these meetings has been substantial. This conference obviously is no exception, judging from the large attendance. Our best wishes for a productive conference.

Raymond M. Rice, M.D.
Vice President, Pharmaceutical Manufacturers Association Foundation, Washington, D.C.

I want to take this opportunity to thank the organizations which have joined together with the Food and Drug Administration (FDA) to support this meeting. The particular interest of the FDA in this conference derives from one of our important responsibilities – namely assuring uniform quality of the nation's drug supply. For many years the FDA has maintained programs aimed at insuring that all drugs meet the standards set by our official compendia, the USP and the National Formulary (NF). These programs include the certification of antibiotics and insulin, the surveillance of selected drugs of particular medical importance by the National Center for Drug Analyses in St. Louis, and the spot checking of selected drug products in our 17 field laboratories.

If we are to assure the medical profession and patients that every formulation of a given drug is safe and effective, we must have objective criteria for determining the equivalency of similar drug products produced by different manufacturers. The problem has been expressed most succinctly by *A.H. Beckett,* a Bristish pharmaceutical scientist, who said '... a drug is not given to man: what is given is a preparation containing the drug'. Certainly one of the important objective methods for evaluating a drug preparation and establishing its equivalency to a referenced drug is bioavailability. The time has passed when chemical equivalency can be considered the sole criterion of acceptability by a manufacturer for marketing a drug, the safety and efficacy of whose reference standard has previously been demonstrated in clinical trials.

The word 'bioavailability' is a relatively new one, or at least its widespread usage seems to be new. In our judgment the term deserves a well agreed-upon operational definition. This was brought home to us most recently in an abbreviated new drug application received by the FDA. This particular application under the heading of Biological Availability read as follows: 'This drug is also available in England and in France.' The definition of bioavailability currently followed in our Bureau of Drugs is rather simple and I think straightforward, and we hope it can remain so. To us bioavailability simply means the degree and rate of absorption of a drug as determined by blood levels or urinary excretion rates or by appropriate short term *in vivo* pharmacological studies. It is not meant to include therapeutic equivalence as determined by clinical trials.

The FDA's interest in bioavailability studies as a tool for helping us with regulatory decisions stems from the 1962 amendments of the Food, Drug and Cosmetic Act and from recommendations made by the D-HEW Task Force on Prescription Drugs. This task force was established by the President to undertake a comprehensive study of the problems of including the cost of prescription drugs under 'Medicare'. The issue of drug quality and 'generic equivalency' and their economic implications were an essential part of this review. As you all know, following the enactment of the 1962 amendments to the Act, the agency contracted with the National Academy of Sciences / National Research Council, for a review of the efficacy of drugs marketed between 1938–1962. In implementing the provisions of the Act and of the review, the FDA has frequently requested evidence of the biological availability of marketed drug formulations. The decision to require data on bioavailability arose as a practical alternative to full clinical trials to demonstrate the efficacy in the use of drugs, as required by the amendments.

Although the primary purpose of this conference is, as I understand it, a scientific assessment of the state of the art in bioavailability, I thought you might be interested in knowing FDA's current regulatory position on bioavailability requirements. As a practical matter, we face the problem of assuring the public that all manufacturers of all drugs reviewed under the Drug Efficacy Study produce products which are safe and efficacious. Biological availability data in lieu of clinical trials are, therefore, required for (1) all products suitable for abbreviated new drug applications, providing a methodology is feasible, and (2) for all revised formulations of previously approved drugs (which were originally found effective in clinical trials), again providing methodology is feasible.

At present we accept the results of studies in which single doses of the test drug and of a referenced preparation are compared in an appropriately designed crossover study in a small number of patients. The function measured may be either the concentration of a drug in the blood over an appropriate time period or the urinary excretion of the drug or some relevant pharmacological or physiological response. Suitable statistical analysis of the data are necessary. We are well aware that studies of this type although simple in their conception, raise a number of fundamental questions such as: What preparation should be used as the 'referenced product'? How should we evaluate certain statistically significant differences in blood levels between the test compound and the referenced drug, when in the vast majority of cases there are no data correlating the blood level of the reference drug with its degree of efficacy? Are other factors, such as whether a drug is taken with meals, more important than the pharmaceutical formulation in determining the effective bioavailability when the drug is actually used clinically in patients? As you are well aware, there are no firm answers to these questions which are applicable to every drug preparation. For this reason, bioavailability information relating to a particular drug product is judged on its own merits in determining whether that product can be considered as equivalent to the referenced product. We all recognize that refinements are needed in our decision-making criteria and I am hopeful this conference will help us achieve a firmer set of guide lines on the interpretation of bioavailability data.

Having outlined our general policy, I would now like to comment on certain special cases in which we depart from this general approach. The first special case is that of true solutions intended for intravenous administration. Bioavailability data are not required for such preparations.

A second special case is that of nonabsorbable drugs administered orally when the action is intended to be local. In this case it is necessary to establish that the manufacturing process has not increased the absorbability of the compound and that it is in fact satisfactorily available locally for therapeutic effect. These considerations also apply to topical preparations administered to the skin or mucus membranes. A third special case is drugs administered by injection where the action is intended to be mainly local. In this case it is necessary to establish that the manufacturing process has not increased the rate of absorption and that the drug is satisfactorily available locally. For a number of drug classes, especially a number of topical preparations intended for use on the skin or in the eyes or ears, product equivalency may be established more easily by clinical trials than by bioavailability studies, and this evidence of therapeutic efficacy can be used in support of a modified new drug application.

A final special situation which perhaps deserves comment is the drug intended for oral use for which no suitable analytical method is available for the performance of bioavailability studies. In this case the FDA will make a determination as to whether clinical trials should be performed to establish unequivocally the efficacy of the preparation of whether *in vitro* tests such as dissolution rates will be considered acceptable. This judgment will take into consideration the seriousness of the disease being treated and the importance of assuming adequate therapeutic equivalency in relation to the referenced product.

In outlining this policy, I would like to emphasize that we sincerely hope our current approach is a temporary one and that it can be modified substantially in the future as a result of progress in biopharmaceutical research. The use of bioavailability studies and clinical trials in patients is a cumbersome, slow, and expensive approach to establishing the therapeutic equivalence of two drug preparations. There is a great need for reliable *in vitro* test procedures which can accurately predict the bioavailability of a drug preparation *in vivo*. The FDA already supports a modest contract program in this field, but more research effort on this important topic is clearly needed, and I look to all of the parties represented at this conference – industry, academic, and government – to contribute to the solution of this problem.

Charles C. Edwards, M.D.

Commissioner, Food and Drug Administration, Department of Health, Education and Welfare

Introduction

The Conference and Progress Toward Standards for Bioavailability

The Food and Drug Act recognizes the authority of the *United States Pharmacopeia* to set strength and quality standards for Pharmacopeial drugs and provides for FDA enforcement of these public standards. In fulfilling this responsibility the USP Committee of Revision attempts to set only standards that are reasonable in ensuring the medical efficacy and safety of the product and that are attainable in production.

In tackling the problem of setting standards of bioavailability, then, the Subcommittee on Bioavailability believed it would be helpful to hold a public conference in which the capabilities of testing and control, as well as the perceived need for public standards, could be openly discussed. Subcommittee Chairman *Azarnoff* was also a member of the Drug Research Board of the National Academy of Sciences/National Research Council. He suggested that the Board be asked to cosponsor the conference. It is believed that a wider audience was reached and that researchers achieved a greater degree of understanding of the potential for setting legal standards in this area to take advantage of advances revealed by recent research.

The Conference, as a conference, was acknowledged a success. The experts had their say, the audience had their questions. Reducing the words to writing has been slow, however: these Proceedings have taken three times longer than promised – and the USP Subcommittee on Bioavailability has yet to expose to public scrutiny and criticism the first proposal for a bioavailability standard for any drug. Nevertheless, the implications of the Conference are clear.

(1) For some drug products, confidence that they have a desired, reproducible medical performance is dependent on the establishment of *public* standards of bioavailability.

(2) The freedom to produce formulations with different medical performances is dependent on *public* standards of bioavailability so that physicians and pharmacists can understand the labeled distinctions between different formulations of the same drug dosage form and use the one most advantageous to the individual patient.

USP is a broad voluntary system operated by the professions of medicine and pharmacy. Those who read these Proceedings and are inspired to offer help in any way are invited to write to the USP Director of Revision, Dr. *Thomas J. Macek.*

William M. Heller
Executive Director
United States Pharmacopeial Convention, Inc.

Pharmacology *8:* 17–20 (1972)

The Rationale for the Conference

F.D. Lawrason
University of Texas Southwestern Medical School, Dallas, Tex.

For many years the physician and the pharmacist have proceeded on the assumption that except in extraordinary instances, a drug once absorbed from either the gastrointestinal tract or the muscle is available to the body for whatever pharmacologic action it might command. However, at the same time it was fully recognized that some drugs appeared to be more effective than others and that this inequality might be due in part to a differential in the so-called bioavailability of the drug. Since biological availability hinges in part on absorption, if there is any question in the physician's mind about absorption of the drug he might simply double the dosage to assure a therapeutic effect. Indeed, there are a few classical drugs such as digitalis which were given in such dosage ranges as to carry their pharmacologic effect to toxicity and then retreat to what was assumed to be an optimal therapeutic effect without overt side effects.

During these many years of therapeutic groping and uncertainty, the physician could not but help to equate dosage with effectiveness and indeed this is for the most part the universal guide line used in the practice of medicine today. Accordingly, for all practical purposes, as one deals with the multiplicity of variables and uncertainties in human pharmacology, it must be recognized that this is not a bad guide line for the physician even though much of the time he either over or under treats his patients in his daily practice.

However, as new scientific knowledge and techniques are acquired and new competence and medical sophistication are attained, one can no longer be satisfied solely with assumptions regarding optimal treatment which is not supported by firm scientific data.

This brings us to the question facing us at this conference. Are we at the stage where there are sound adequate scientific data regarding the biological availability of drugs to support new pharmacologic and therapeutic guide lines for the physician? Proof of bioavailability is being requested and indeed demanded for both new and duplicate-type drugs by the Food and Drug Administration (FDA). This is not an unreasonable request for it does not really entail anything new about what has been requested over the past ten or more years. It involves the same basic parameters as studied in the past: absorption, metabolism, and excretion. These represent fundamental data that should be gathered and confirmed for any drug.

At the same time, it should be understood that such data cannot be equated with efficacy except by inference. They merely quantitate to the best of our knowledge and techniques, rates of absorption, blood levels and their duration, and identify the metabolic pathways as well as rates of excretion by whatever route. From such data, one should be able to arrive at a dosage regimen which in turn will lead to pharmacologic and therapeutic ranges of effectiveness and safety. These latter two end points, effectiveness and safety, are in the final analysis, the therapeutic objectives in the use of drugs of medicine. Efficacy and safety of any drug must be based on the best possible scientific data available, but it must be remembered that the bioavailability of a drug in the circulation is but one important step to this end.

It is obvious that if bioavailability is to be meaningful, and supportive to both the investigator and to the practitioner, appropriate tests and techniques must be carried out *in vivo* in the human. It is possible that *in vitro* tests at times may be more accurate and discriminating and can give substantial insight, guidance and clues for predictive purposes, as a drug is carried through preliminary studies. Solubility and dissolution rates are important in the preparation and control of a drug and may indeed correlate closely with the ultimate *in vivo* tests for bioavailability. However, even if there is a close correlation between the *in vitro* and *in vivo* data, the final proof of biological availability must rest solidly on sound scientific *in vivo* data. In the instance of a close correlation between *in vitro* and *in vivo* data, proper standards could be established which may be most helpful and reassuring for purposes of a continuing basis of surveillance.

Similarly, there is no question that *in vivo* animal tests and experiments involving bioavailability are basic to the development of a new drug. However, once safety has been established on a preliminary basis in animals, the proof of biological availability in man rests only in man himself. To my knowledge, there is no convincing evidence nor are there data reflecting bioavailability in animals which can in any way transcend or substitute for data collected in man. Thus, it is of paramount importance that accurate bioassays of a given compound be established early in the development of a new drug. Only in this way, can a proper dosage regimen based on scientific data be established. At the same time, evidence of therapeutic effectiveness can begin to be equated with blood levels and their duration. Similarly, perhaps some insight can be gained and significant correlations made involving blood levels leading to important data concerning the safety of the drug.

Isotopically labeled compounds have given solid evidence of the presence of drugs in various tissues, but except in certain instances, it is not possible to quantitate these data at either a pharmacologic or therapeutic level. For the most part, radioactively labeled material is most effectively used in studying metabolic pathways, tissue deposition and ultimate rates of excretion. Here again, assay of total radioactivity cannot substitute for accurate biochemical methods of assay. Thus, even though labeled material does provide clues of bioavailability, they do not carry substantive and definitive proof.

From what has been said and what will be said further at this conference, the study of the pharmacokinetics involved with the biological and medical issues of bioavailability are extremely complicated. I am not at all sure that one can entirely equate the pharmacologic or therapeutic performance of a drug with its biological availability as we think of it today. Obviously, if a drug is effective in carrying out its designed therapeutic task, it can be assumed that it was available to the body biologically. On the other hand, if it fails to be effective, it cannot be simply assumed that it was not available in sufficient amounts in the blood stream.

All of us are well acquainted with the curious variations of responsiveness from patient to patient to almost every drug. Blood levels, duration, and excretion rates may be entirely within the usual range of therapeutic effectiveness for that particular drug, yet there is hardly a drug available today that is 100-percent predictive with regard to effectiveness. Perhaps the antibiotics as a general class of drugs conform the best in this regard and even these have their problems.

The human as a species is perhaps the most highly complicated biological hybrid known, and I suspect that until we go beyond the simple bioavailability of a drug within the circulation and penetrate into the target of diseased and injured tissues of the body, many of the these therapeutic dilemmas will persist. Of course, this effort would take us into entirely new spheres or levels of biochemical sophistication and technical know-how that is unavailable today. Thus, with the exception of a few diseases where some technical inroads have been made, it is essential that scientific clarification and understanding be reached on the basis of presently known knowledge on the biological availability of drugs before moving aimlessly into the target tissues beyond the blood stream.

As all of us know, there are a multiplicity of physiological and biological factors which have both direct and indirect bearing on the absorption and biological availability of a drug. With each new drug, there is an earnest attempt on the part of the research team first studying the drug to define these factors as precisely as possible. However, more frequently than not, it is only after broad experience that the physician can be given the proper guide lines under which to administer the drug in order to bring the greatest degree of effectiveness and safety to his patients.

This conference is designed to explore known scientific data and techniques used in the evaluation of the bioavailability of drugs, to reveal present limitations in these techniques, and to place in perspective the issue of the degree of importance as well as the essentials that can be placed on the meaning of the term bioavailability at this point in time. Any discussion during this conference directed at any particular drug must not be misconstrued as an individual reflection or shortcoming of that particular drug, but merely as an example of the problem or problems faced in the study of all drugs. Everyone participating in this conference must recognize that in order to grapple with some of these problems, one must deal with specifics, and it is for this reason that as certain topics are discussed, certain examples involving specific drugs will be cited in order to quantitate facts and figures and arrive at whatever conclusions can be made with regard to present knowledge on bioavailability. These should be merely treated as case histories and nothing else.

Thus, it is the sincere hope of the program committee and the sponsoring organizations that this conference will be open, informal and thoughtful as well as forthright, and anything said by way of specifics during these two days will not be misconstrued as a shortcoming or limitation directed at any agency, company or drug. We hope the conference will be constructive in increasing our present knowledge as well as our limitations, the scientific needs and perhaps the direction that must be pursued if we are to advance on a more sound scientific basis in this important field.

In my opinion, if we are to pursue these goals successfully, a broadly based cooperative effort must be developed involving the laboratories and clinical facilities of the universities and their medical centers, the pharmaceutical laboratories and the efforts and understanding of the federal agencies and independent organizations, such as the USP, and the Drug Research Board of the National Academy of Sciences as well as other research groups. Without this kind of cooperation and understanding among all those concerned, we cannot expect real progress in the field of drug research and medical therapeutics.

Once again, it is our sincere hope that this conference will in some part stimulate new ideas, concepts and efforts which will be constructive in bringing some of these problems into sharper focus based on a more firm foundation of sound scientific data.

Author's address: Dr. *F. Douglas Lawrason*, University of Texas Southwestern Medical School, 5323 Harry Hines Boulevard, *Dallas, TX 75235* (USA)

Pharmacology *8:* 21–32 (1972)

Mechanisms of Drug Absorption and of Drug Solution

D.J. Jollow and B.B. Brodie

Laboratory of Chemical Pharmacology, National Heart and Lung Institute, National Institutes of Health, Bethesda, Md.

As recently described by *Hogben* (12), the gastrointestinal barrier is structurally a complex assemblage of lipids, proteins, lipoproteins and polysaccharides. It may be regarded as an extended sheath of epithelial cells so closely packed that they form a virtually continuous lipoidal boundary. Lipid-soluble substances penetrate the gastrointestinal boundary through passive diffusion by dissolving in the lipid-like phase; polar substances also penetrate by passive diffusion if, like ethanol, urea and water, they are small enough to filter through microscopic 'pores' in the membrane or through the spaces between the cells. The gastrointestinal membrane also possesses a number of specialized transport mechanisms for nutrients such as amino acids, sugars, purines, pyrimidines and vitamins.

The Nature of the Absorption Process

The question arises whether drugs pass through the gastrointestinal membrane by passive diffusion or by means of specialized transport mechanisms. If a drug is absorbed by a specialized transport mechanism, it should saturate the process at high concentrations and its absorption should be inhibited by structurally similar drugs. For most drugs, the proportional rates of drug absorption in the rat intestine are unchanged over a very wide range of drug concentrations and these rates are not decreased by the presence of structurally similar drugs. It seems unlikely, therefore, that therapeutic agents, unless they are structurally similar to normal nutrients (e.g. antimetabolites) are absorbed from the gastrointestinal tract by specialized transport mechanisms (13, 14, 30, 31).

If drugs are absorbed by passive diffusion through a lipoid membrane, their rate of absorption should depend on their solubility in the lipoidal membrane.

Table I. Comparison between colonic absorption and lipid-to-water partition of the unionized forms of barbiturates[1]

	Percent absorbed[2]	Chloroform-to-water partition coefficient
Barbital	12	0.7
Apobarbital	17	4.9
Phenobarbital	20	4.8
Allylbarbituric acid	23	10.5
Butethal	24	11.7
Cyclobarbital	24	13.9
Pentobarbital	30	28.0
Secobarbital	40	50.7
Hexethal	44	>100

1 From *Schanker* (29).

2 Percent change of concentration of drug in saline perfused for 20 min at 0.2 ml/min through the entire colon.

The validity of this concept is illustrated in table I which compares the rates of colonic absorption of a variety of barbiturates with their chloroform/water partition coefficients (29). Variation in the degree of ionization of the drugs was not a factor in this study since the nine barbiturates tested are essentially nonionized at the pH (6.8) of the solution in the colon. The data show that the absorption rates of the barbiturates are roughly proportional to their lipid solubility. Using the small intestine, *Hogben et al.* (14) showed a similar correlation between intestinal absorption and lipid solubility for a variety of basic and acid drugs. The absorption of drug structures as diverse as phenylbutazone, acetylsalicylic acid and sulfanilamide showed the same dependence on lipid solubility. It should be noted that the correlations are of rank order only. The difficulty in demonstrating a more exact correlation lies in the use of organic solvents to assess 'lipid solubility' of drugs in the gastrointestinal membrane. The use of the chloroform/water partition coefficient to predict penetration through the lipoidal membrane has been experimentally valuable, but it is obviously not a perfect model. *Hogben* (12) has suggested that future studies might profitably employ a lipid phase consisting of cholesterol and phospholipids in the same proportions in which they occur in the erythrocyte membrane.

The pH Partition Theory

The difficulty in demonstrating that the absorption of drugs is essentially a process of passive diffusion through a lipoid membrane is the fact that they are usually organic electrolytes which may be only partially undissociated at physiological pHs. Our understanding of the interrelationships between the rate of drug absorption, the dissociation constant (pKa) and the pH of the absorption site is known as the *pH-partition theory* (33). This theory, which is based on extensive investigations (13, 14, 30, 31, 33), states that the passage of drugs across the gastrointestinal barrier is restricted to the undissociated drug form; therefore the rate of absorption depends on the proportion of drug present in this form. In other words, the rate of absorption depends not only on the lipid solubility of the drug, but on its degree of ionization; the latter in turn is a function of the pKa and the pH of the absorbing surface.

Table II compares the relation between the degree of ionization and the relative rates of absorption from the stomach of a number of acids and bases of widely different chemical structure (30). A strong acid (e.g. 5-sulfosalicyclic acid) whose pKa value is below 1 is completely ionized even in the acid contents of the stomach and shows little absorption. Weaker acids, such as salicylic and 5-nitrosalicylic acid, are largely undissociated at pH 1 and are appreciably absorbed. At this pH, weak bases are highly ionized and are absorbed only negligibly. More direct evidence for the view that only the undissociated drug form is absorbed is supplied by changes in drug absorption when gastric juice is replaced with bicarbonate solution (pH 8). Acids like salicylic and nitrosalicylic are absorbed much more poorly since neutralization of the gastric acidity de-

Table II. Comparison of gastric absorption at pH 1 and 8 in the rat[1]

	pKa	Absorption at pH 1, %[2]	Absorption at pH 8, %
Acids			
5-Sulfosalicylic	strong	0	0
5-Nitrosalicylic	2.3	52	16
Salicylic	3.0	61	13
Thiopental	7.6	46	34
Phenol	9.9	40	40
Bases			
Aniline	4.6	6	56
p-Toluidine	5.3	0	47
Quinine	8.4	0	18
Dextrorphan	9.2	0	16
Procaine amide ethobromide	strong	0	0

1 From *Schanker et al.* (30).

2 One hour absorption of 1 mg of drug in 5 ml of 0.1 N HCl, or in 5 ml of pH 8 buffer.

creases the concentration of the lipid-soluble undissociated forms. The same pH change does not appreciably affect very weak acids like thiopental and phenol since even at pH 8 they remain almost wholly undissociated. Conversely, neutralizing the stomach contents causes a substantial increase in the absorption of weak bases by increasing the concentration of the undissociated form. The quaternary cations are not absorbed at either pH.

It may be inferred from these results that acidic but not basic drugs are absorbed directly from the stomach. As shown in figure 1, weak acids such as salicylic, thiopental and aspirin, are readily absorbed from the stomach of the human whereas bases, such as aminopyrine and ephedrine, are not (13). Very weakly basic drugs (pKa < 2.5) such as antipyrine are absorbed from the stomach to some extent since they are significantly nonionized at pH 1.

Similar evidence shows that the pH-partition theory also applies to the absorption of drugs from the small intestine (31). Table III shows the relative rates for a considerable number of acids and bases. The weak acids, those with a pKa of 3 or higher, are absorbed relatively rapidly; the acids of intermediate strength (pKa 2.2 to 2.9) are absorbed more slowly and the completely ionized acids were absorbed hardly at all. Similarly the weak bases, those of pKa below 8.4 are in general absorbed relatively rapidly, the bases of intermediate strength, those with a pKa between 8.4 and 11 are absorbed more slowly; and the completely ionized quaternary ammonium compounds are absorbed hardly at all.

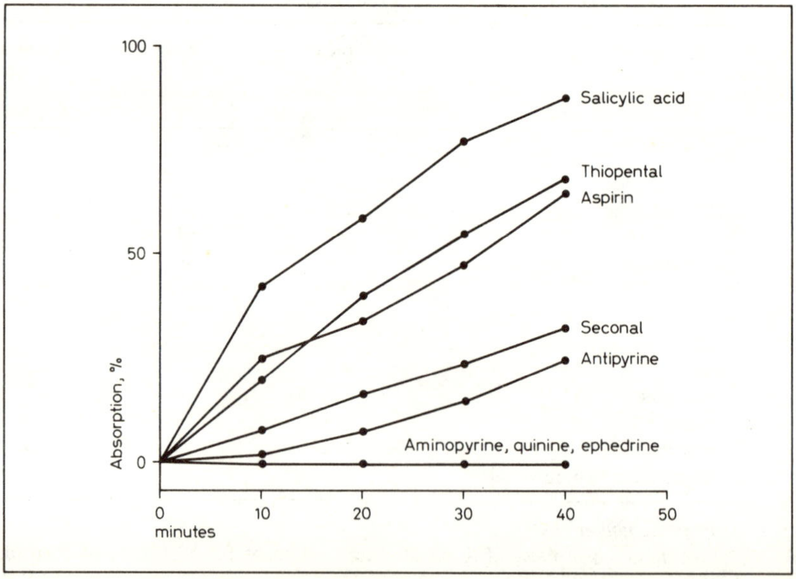

Fig. 1. Relative rates of drug absorption from the human stomach. From *Hogben et al.* (13).

Table III. Absorption of drugs from small intestine of rats[1]

Acids	pKa	Absorption[2]	Bases	pKa	Absorption[2]
5-Sulfosalicylic	strong	< 2	Acetanilide	0.3	42
Phenol red	strong	< 2	Theophylline	0.7	29
Bromphenol blue	strong	< 2	*p*-Nitroaniline	1.0	68
o-Nitrobenzoic	2.2	5	Antipyrine	1.4	32
5-Nitrosalicylic	2.3	9	*m*-Nitroaniline	2.5	77
Tromexan	2.9	35	Aniline	4.6	54
Salicylic	3.0	60	Aminopyrine	5.0	33
m-Nitrobenzoic	3.4	53	*p*-Toluidine	5.3	59
Acetylsalicylic	3.5	20	Quinine	8.4	15
Benzoic	4.2	51	Ephedrine	9.6	7
Phenylbutazone	4.4	65	Tolazoline	10.3	6
Acetic	4.7	42	Mecamylamine	11.2	3
Thiopental	7.6	55	Darstine	strong	< 2
Barbital	7.8	30	Procaine amide ethobromide	strong	< 2
p-Hydroxypropiophenone	7.8	61	Tetraethylammonium	strong	< 2
Phenol	9.9	51	Tensilon	strong	< 2

1 From *Schanker et al.* (31).
2 Percent change of concentration of drug in saline perfused for 7 min at 1.5 ml/min through the entire small intestine. Zero absorption indicates that absorption is too slow to be measured by this method.

The observation that the weak acids and bases are absorbed more readily than the stronger, highly ionized acids and bases suggests that the barrier separating the intestinal lumen from blood is preferentially permeable to the undissociated forms of drugs. This concept is sustained by the observed rates of absorption of a number of drugs from solutions of different pH (14). If the concept is valid, the absorption of a drug should be enhanced by a change in the pH that increases the proportion of the undissociated moiety. And so as the pH of the intestine is decreased, acids are absorbed better, and bases more poorly. In contrast, as the pH is increased, bases are absorbed better, and acids more poorly (14). These results indicate that gastric and intestinal absorption are similar in nature. Hence variation in absorption rates of organic acids and bases in different parts of the gastrointestinal tract reflect differences in pH of the lumen and are not due to different processes.

One point still to be settled is the pH at the membrane surface of the mucosa, since this would determine the actual proportion of undissociated drug and therefore the rate of absorption. An indication that the pH at the absorptive surface is not the same as that of the bulk intestinal contents is found in table III which shows that in the normal intestine, acids with pKa > 3 and bases with pKa < 7.8 are well absorbed; outside these limits the absorption of acids and bases, respectively, fall off rapidly. Accepting the pH of the intestinal fluids as 6.5, calculation shows that the proportion of nonionized molecules would be 1:5,000 for acids and 1:15 for bases. This difference in permeability of the nonionized forms is not in accordance with the concept of a lipoid boundary since it would imply a greater permeability to the nonionized form of acids than to that of bases. A simpler possibility would be that the actual resorptive surface is bathed by a fluid with a pH of less than 6.5.

This point was settled by simultaneously perfusing drugs intravenously and through the intestine. If the intestinal absorption of drugs is simply a matter of diffusion of the unionized drug moiety across a lipoidal barrier, it should be possible to calculate the pH of the absorbing surface from the plasma/lumen concentration ratio at the steady state (14). The pH of the absorbing surface was calculated to be 5.3, a value consistent with the finding that the intestinal mucosa secretes hydrogen ions (5, 14). A pH of 5.3 would explain why the lowest pKa of an acidic drug compatible with rapid absorption is about 3, while the corresponding pKa for bases is about 8. Given a pH of 5.3 at the absorbing surface, the proportion of nonionized to ionized drug necessary for rapid absorption is 1:300 both for an acid of pKa 2.8 and for a base of pKa 7.8.

Whatever the precise nature of the absorption of foreign compounds from the gastrointestinal tract, it is possible to formulate a number of general rules based on the principles discussed above. Organic electrolytes should be readily absorbed from solution in the small intestine if the undissociated form has a favorable chloroform to water partition, and if the pKa for an acid is greater than 2 and for a base is less than 10. Also, acidic drugs will be absorbed from solution in the stomach if the pKa is greater than 2.

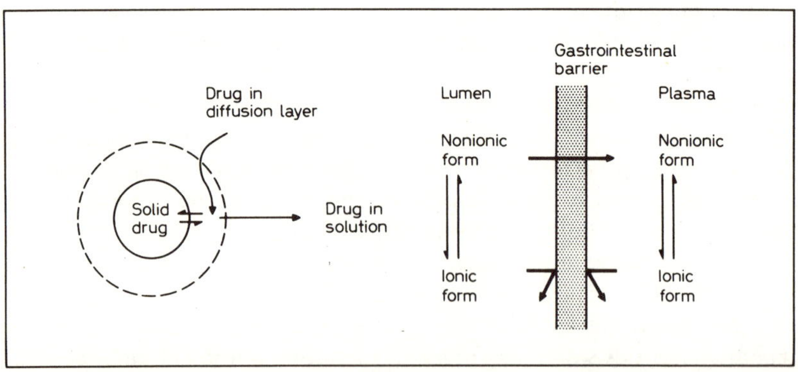

Fig. 2. Schematic representation of the relationship between a solid drug in the lumen and the absorption process.

Importance of Solubility in the Bioavailability of Drugs

The studies, discussed above, were carried out on drugs in solution so that by definition, permeability in the intestinal membrane is the rate-limiting step in absorption. For many drugs, however, absorption is limited by poor solubility at the pH of the gastrointestinal tract. The rate-limiting step in absorption now becomes the rate at which the solid drug enters the bulk solution (fig. 2). This can be true even with drugs that have a high chloroform/water partition coefficient. Dissolution-limited absorption may occur even if the drug is given as a water-soluble salt. For example, a sodium salt may precipitate as the free acid in the gastric juice.

The importance of solubility in limiting the rate of absorption is seen with phenylbutazone analogues. Several of these analogues given parenterally to rats are highly active in protecting against formaldehyde-induced edema, but are almost devoid of action when given orally to man. This was the result of poor absorption, for low plasma levels were obtained after oral administration compared to high levels when the drugs were given intravenously. In table IV is shown the relative solubility of phenylbutazone and a number of its analogues. Those with solubilities > 1.5 mg/ml were well absorbed while those with solu-

Table IV. Comparison of solubilities of phenylbutazone analogues at pH 7 with their oral absorption[1]

Compound	Structure	Solubility mg/ml at pH 7	Absorption after oral administration to man
	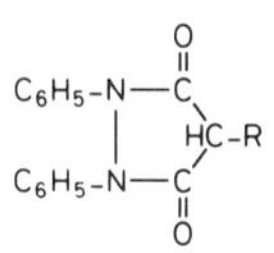		
Phenylbutazone	$R = CH_2CH_2CH_2CH_3$	2.2	rapid and complete
Metabolite 1	$R = CH_2CH_2CH_2CH_3$	10	rapid and complete
G-1	$R = CH_2CH_2SC_6H_5$	1.6	rapid and complete
G-3	$R = CH_2CH_2CH_2C_6H_5$	0.14	slow and incomplete
G-8	$R = CH_2CH_2SC_6H_3$ o,p, $(CH_3)_2$	0.13	slow and incomplete
G-20	$R = CH_2CH_2CH_2CH_3$	0.09	slow and incomplete
G-21	$R = CH_2CH_2CH_2CH_3$	0.12	slow and incomplete
G-23	$R = \overset{O}{\overset{\|}{C}}\text{-}CH_2CH_2CH_3$	0.12	slow and incomplete

1 From *Brodie* (5).

bilities of 0.15 mg/ml or less were poorly absorbed. Actually the *rates* of solution rather than the *degree* of solution should have been compared; the poor oral bioavailability presumably reflects the slow rate of solution in the gut.

The rate and degree of absorption of an orally administered drug is dependent on two different processes, the dissolution characteristics in water and the permeability characteristics across the intestinal membrane. The rate-limiting step for drugs that are soluble at the pH of the small intestine is the rate at which a drug penetrates the intestinal barrier (intrinsic permeability); in contrast, the rate-limiting step for drugs that are relatively insoluble in the small intestine may be the rate at which the solid drug goes into solution (intrinsic dissolution rate).

Emphasis has been placed on the *in vitro* screening for dissolution properties of a drug, but such a test does not appraise the intrinsic permeability in the intestine membrane. For example, quaternary ammonium compounds and guanethidine have a high dissolution rate in the intestinal fluids but are slowly and incompletely absorbed because of poor permeability. In contrast, a drug such as griseofulvin is slowly absorbed despite its high intrinsic permeability because of a very slow rate of dissolution.

Therefore, in addition to testing for dissolution rate, a test is also needed to appraise intrinsic permeability through the intestinal membrane. The permeability characteristics of most therapeutic agents may be obtained by measuring the partition coefficient between chloroform and water buffered to pH 5.3, the calculated pH of the absorbing surface of the small intestine. In general, a partition ratio of 0.5 or greater is consistent with reasonably good intrinsic permeability, but additional research is needed to establish this value. Alternatively, the permeability characteristics may be obtained from the *in situ* perfusion of the rat's small intestine as described by *Hogben et al.* (14). The latter method of testing would include in the category of permeable drugs those polar substances that are absorbed by specialized transport systems. Thus by measuring both intrinsic dissolution and intrinsic permeability of a drug it should be possible to determine whether dissolution or permeability will be a rate-limiting step in absorption.

In drug development, it is important to evaluate the bioavailability of the drug before it is formulated and before clinical trials are attempted. Such tests of dissolution and permeability may well anticipate difficulties in drug absorption and enable proper decisions to be made on which form of the drug should be used in formulation and clinical studies. Although bioavailability studies must finally be carried out in man, it is important in drug development to obtain preliminary assessment of bioavailability in animals. In fact, it is possible that the results of bioavailability studies in large animals, such as dogs (in tests in which each animal is its own control) may be extrapolated to man. In view of the practical difficulties of making large numbers of such measurements in man, additional research is needed to establish whether bioavailability is similar in man and dog.

The importance of measuring the absolute bioavailability cannot be overstressed. The area under the plasma concentration-time curve after oral administration is compared with that after intravenous administration by simply plotting arithmetically the plasma concentration curves of unchanged drug (using each animal as its own control). The investigator now cuts out the areas under the curves and weighs them. The degree of absorption is the ratio of the two weights. In most instances, such comparisons will yield the percentage of drug that is absorbed when given orally.

If the bioavailability of the drug is poor as shown by the area under the curve, the *in vitro* tests mentioned above might serve to show which parameter is at fault, drug-dissolution or drug permeability. If the latter, nothing can be done except to look for a more suitable drug; if the former, attempts can be made to improve the rates of solution by changes in crystal form, micronization, use of surfactants, etc.

Certain precautions are needed in the interpretation of the plasma-level time-course curves. A drug may show by *in vitro* testing all the characteristics for ready absorption yet have a poor bioavailability: (1) If the drug is unstable in the gastrointestinal tract, for example, dibenamine congeners react chemically with material in the gut; (2) certain drugs such as chlorpromazine may be metabolized to a considerable degree by enzymes in the intestinal mucosa; (3) a drug may be metabolized so rapidly by liver enzymes that the rate constant of elimination approaches that of absorption. This results in the so-called first-pass effects in which a major part of the drug is changed in its passage through the liver. Among such drugs are glyceryl trinitrate which has little effect when taken by stomach but is very effective when absorbed sublingually.

Brief mention shall be made of some of the techniques used to overcome dissolution-limited absorption. These include the use of sodium, potassium, or calcium salts of acidic drugs, micronization of the solid crystals, solubilization by surfactants, and the use of anhydrous, amorphous, or metastable crystalline forms of the drugs.

Salt forms are believed to increase the rate of solution of the solid drug by providing a buffer layer of pH higher than that of gastric juice around the crystal surface. In fact, similar increased dissolution rates have been obtained when the solid acid form of the drug was compounded together with a trisodium phosphate buffer (25). Salt forms have been used to overcome dissolution-limited absorption for barbiturates (1, 25), sulfonamides (25), novobiocin (7), penicillin V (17), and tolbutamide (26). Perhaps the best known example, or at least the best advertised, is aspirin, which is commonly formulated as the calcium salt or alternatively compounded in the presence of a buffer. Reduction in particle size of the drug crystals (micronization), with consequent increase in the surface area of the crystals exposed to the gastric juice, has been reported to increase the oral availability of sulfadiazine (28) and griseofulvin (2). The use of amorphous and metastable crystalline forms of drugs to increase the absorption of novobiocin (24) and methylprednisolone (3) may be rationalized on the basis of the drug molecules having a greater tendency to leave an energetically less stable lattice structure.

Reduced particle size, and perhaps amorphous structure, presumably underline the increased absorption rate obtained when weakly acidic drugs are administered as aqueous solutions of the sodium or potassium salts. The salts would precipitate rapidly on contact with the highly acidic gastric juice and hence the acid form of the drug would be present as finely dispersed microcrystalline structures or perhaps as amorphous aggregates. A related technique is to disperse the poorly soluble drug in a highly water-soluble solid carrier (e.g. as a melt). On exposure to the gastric juice, the water-soluble material dissolves rapidly, leaving extremely finely divided drug particles (9, 10, 11).

Surfactants have been reported to increase the absorption of sulfisoxazole (18), secobarbital (22), griseofulvin (4), and hexestrol (4), presumably by dissolving the water-insoluble drug in the hydrophobic interior of the surfactant micelle. Dissolution could thus be promoted by either an increased 'wetting' of the drug by the gastric juice or by precipitation of the drug as a fine dispersion on subsequent disruption of the surfactant micelle. It should be noted that surfactants have also been reported to decrease absorption of some drugs including nystatin, polymyxin and vancomycin (32).

Physiological Factors Affecting Absorption

The time of onset of therapeutic effect of drugs which are optimally absorbed from the intestine depends on the rate at which the drug leaves the stomach and enters the duodenum. A variety of biological variables, such as gastric emptying time, intestinal mobility and gastrointestinal contents, may drastically influence the time and rate of absorption. These biological variables are dependent, in turn, on a large number of factors, such as whether the patient is fasted or fed (15, 19, 20), the temperature of the meal (16), the nature of the diet and, in particular, the fat content of the meal (21, 27), and even the posture of a bedridden patient (8). These variables may be of major significance in the oral availability of drugs that are only fractionally available (such as griseofulvin), that are administered in sustained release preparations, that undergo extensive degradation in the gastric juice (such as benzpenicillin), or that irritate the gastric lining on prolonged exposure.

One drug may interfere with the absorption of another. The absorption of certain drugs, especially those that are relatively insoluble in the intestine, may be decreased by drugs that depress the motility of the gastrointestinal tract (6). For example, desipramine lowers the absorption of phenylbutazone (6), presumably by decreasing gastrointestinal motility and thereby lowering the rate of dissolution of the phenylbutazone crystals. Similar effects on gastric emptying and hence drug absorption have been suggested for anticholinergic drugs and for acetaminophen and aspirin (34). Antacid preparations (as well as milk products) have been reported to decrease tetracycline absorption (27) by formation of chelates.

References

1 *Anderson, K.W.:* Oral absorption of quinalbarbitone and its sodium salt. Arch. int. Pharmacodyn. *147:* 171 (1964).

2 *Atkinson, R.M.; Bedford, C.B.; Child, K.J., and Tomich, E.G.:* Effect of particle size on blood griseofulvin levels in man. Nature, Lond. *193:* 588 (1962).

3 *Ballard, B.E. and Nelson, E.:* Physicochemical properties of drugs that control absorption rate after subcutaneous implantation. J. Pharmacol. exp. Ther. *135:* 120 (1962).

4 *Bates, T.; Gibaldi, M., and Kanig, J.L.:* Rate of dissolution of griseofulvin and hexestrol in bile salt solutions. Nature, Lond. *210:* 1331 (1966).

5 *Brodie, B.B.:* Physicochemical factors in drug absorption; in *Binns* Absorption and distribution of drugs, pp. 16–48 (Livingstone, Edinburgh 1964).

6 *Consolo, S. and Garattini, S.:* Effect of desipramine on intestinal absorption of phenylbutazone and other drugs. Europ. J. Pharmacol. *6:* 332 (1969).

7 *Furez, S.:* Blood levels following oral administration of different preparations of novobiocin. Antibiot. Chemother., N.Y. *8:* 448 (1958).

8 *Gibaldi, M. and Kanig, J.L.:* Effect of body positions and pH on gastrointestinal absorption of salicylate and creatinine in man. Arch. int. Pharmacodyn. *161:* 343 (1966).

9 *Goldberg, A.H.; Gibaldi, M., and Kanig, J.L.:* Increasing dissolution rates via solid solutions and eutetic mixtures. I. Theoretical considerations. J. pharm. Sci. *54:* 1145 (1965).

10 *Goldberg, A.H.; Gibaldi, M., and Kanig, J.L.:* Increasing dissolution rates via solid solutions and eutetic mixtures. III. Griseofulvin-succinic acid solid solution. J. pharm. Sci. *55:* 487 (1966).

11 *Goldberg, A.H.; Gibaldi, M.; Kanig, J.L., and Mayersohn, M.:* Increasing dissolution rates via solid solutions and eutetic mixtures. IV. Chloramphenicol-urea system. J. pharm. Sci. *55:* 581 (1966).

12 *Hogben, C.A.M.:* Biological membranes and their passage by drugs; in *Brodie and Gillette* Concepts in biochemical pharmacology, vol. XXVIII, part 1, pp. 1–6 (Springer, New York 1971).

13 *Hogben, C.A.M.; Schanker, L.S.; Tocco, D.J., and Brodie, B.B.:* Absorption of drugs from the stomach. II. The human. J. Pharmacol. exp. Ther. *120:* 540 (1957).

14 *Hogben, C.A.M.; Tocco, D.J.; Brodie, B.B., and Schanker, L.S.:* On the mechanism of intestinal absorption of drugs. J. Pharmacol. exp. Ther. *125:* 275 (1958).

15 *Hunt, J.N.:* Gastric emptying and secretion in man. Physiol. Rev. *39:* 491 (1959).

16 *Hunt, J.N. and Spurrel, W.R.:* Pattern of emptying of the human stomach. J. Physiol., Lond. *113:* 157 (1951).

17 *Juncker, H. and Raaschou, F.:* Solubility of oral preparations of penicillin V. Antibiot. Med. *4:* 497 (1957).

18 *Kakemi, K.; Arita, T., and Muramishi, S.:* Absorption and excretion of drugs. XXVII. Effect of nonionic surfactants on rectal absorption of sulfonamides. Chem. pharm. Bull. *13:* 976 (1965).

19 *Klein, J.O. and Finland, M.:* The new penicillins. New Engl. J. Med. *269:* 1019 (1963).

20 *Kirby, W.M.M.; Roberts, C.E., and Bardick, R.E.:* Comparison of two new tetracyclines with tetracyclines and demethylchlortetracycline. Antimicrobiol. Agents chemother., p. 286 (1961).

21 *Levy, G. and Jusko, W.:* Effect of viscosity on drug absorption. J. pharm. Sci. *54:* 219 (1965).

22 *Levy, G.; Miller, K.E., and Reuning, R.H.:* Effect of complex formation on drug absorption. III. Concentration and drug dependent effect of a nonionic surfactant. J. pharm. Sci. *55:* 394 (1966).

23 *McMartin, C. and Simpson, P.:* The absorption and metabolism of guanethidine in hypertensive patients requiring different doses of the drug. Clin. Pharmacol. Ther. *12:* 73 (1971).

24 *Mullins, J.D. and Macek, T.J.:* Some pharmaceutical properties of novobiocin. J. amer. pharm. Ass. *49:* 245 (1960).

25 *Nelson, E.J.:* Comparative dissolution rates of weak acids and their sodium salts. J. amer. pharm. Ass. *47:* 297 (1958).

26 *Nelson, E.; Knoechel, E.L.; Hamlin, W.E., and Wagner, J.G.:* Influence of absorption rate of tolbutamide on rate of decline of blood sugar levels in normal humans. J. pharm. Sci. *51:* 509 (1962).

27 *Price, K.E.; Zolli, Z.; Atkinson, J.C., and Luther, H.G.:* Antibiotic inhibitors. Antibiot. Chemother. *7:* 672 (1957).

28 *Reinhold, J.G.; Phillips, F.J., and Flippen, H.J.:* Comparison of behavior of microcrystalline sulfadiazine with that of ordinary sulfadiazine in man. Amer. J. med. Sci. *210:* 141 (1945).

29 *Schanker, L.S.:* Absorption of drugs from the rat colon. J. Pharmacol. exp. Ther. *126:* 283 (1959).

30 *Schanker, L.S.; Shore, P.A.; Brodie, B.B., and Hogben, C.A.M.:* Absorption of drugs from the stomach. I. The rat. J. Pharmacol. exp. Ther. *120:* 528 (1957).

31 *Schanker, L.S.; Tocco, D.J.; Brodie, B.B., and Hogben, C.A.M.:* Absorption of drugs from the rat small intestine. J. Pharmacol. exp. Ther. *123:* 81 (1958).

32 *Schneierson, S.S. and Amsterdam, D.:* Effect of bile salts on the activity of antibiotics. Nature, Lond. *182:* 56 (1958).

33 *Shore, P.A.; Brodie, B.B., and Hogben, C.A.M.:* Gastric secretion of drugs – a pH partition hypothesis. J. Pharmacol. exp. Ther. *119:* 361 (1957).

34 *Weikel, J.H. and Lish, P.M.:* Gastrointestinal pharmacology antipyreticanalgetic agents. II. Absorption and smooth muscle effects. Arch. int. Pharmacodyn. *119:* 398 (1959).

Authors' address: Dr. *David J. Jollow* and Dr. *Bernard B. Brodie*, Laboratory of Chemical Pharmacology, National Heart and Lung Institute, National Institutes of Health, *Bethesda, MD 20014* (USA)

Pharmacology *8:* 33–43 (1972)

Bioavailability, Clinical Effectiveness, and the Public Interest

G. Levy

Department of Pharmaceutics, School of Pharmacy, State University of New York at Buffalo, N.Y.

We have come together at this meeting specifically to consider problems related to the bioavailability of drugs but, in broader terms, we are in effect addressing ourselves to the question of how we can provide the public with drugs of high quality at reasonable cost within the framework of our free enterprise system. Free enterprise in the area of health care requires a particularly high level of individual and corporate responsibility or the privileges of freedom that we value so highly will soon be eroded. The public expects, and rightfully so, that we in the health sciences and health professions adhere to standards of performance and ethics which are higher than average. If we act selfishly, if we fail to perform in a manner consistent with the public interest, then our professions and our industries will become subject to an increasing number of constraints and impositions by government acts in response to public demand. This would be unfortunate, not only for us in the field of health care, but even more so for our nation, in that it would serve notice that our way of life and our concepts of individual freedom and free enterprise are not compatible with the provision of high-quality health care to the public.

The fact that we have gathered here to direct our combined efforts and competences toward the development of higher standards of drug product performance, to assure to the best of our ability their quality and safety, is evidence that we can and will carry out our responsibilities. For much more than a century, physicians and pharmacists have worked together, on their own initiative and without government or public prompting, to assure that our drugs are of the highest quality. We can proudly point to the fact that our official standards of drug quality, as represented by the USP and National Formulary, are not the result of governmental edict but derive solely from the efforts and sense of responsibility of the health professions. Only we in the US can make this claim.

The Need for Bioavailability Testing

Those who preceded us in the development of drug standards responded to needs and problems in accordance with their experience and knowledge. When one and the same drug was prescribed and labeled by different names in different parts of the country, or by individuals with different academic background, our predecessors standardized drug nomenclature. When impurities or degradation products presented a problem, they imposed limits on these. They developed tests to assure the identity of drugs, and assay methods to assess potency. They established limits of potency so that tablets labeled as containing a given amount of drug did indeed contain that amount within reasonably narrow limits. When it became apparent more recently that tablets or capsules satisfied these limits on the average (when ten or more units are assayed together) but not individually, the potency tests were refined further in that individual dosage units have to be analyzed and are required to conform to defined standards. The purpose of all these standards and tests was to make sure that the patient, when taking a prescribed medication, receives exactly the dose prescribed, within the defined limits. When digitalis tablets were thought to contain up to 10 % more than the amount of drug designated by the USP, and warfarin tablets were suspected to deviate 6–8 % from label claim, then these products were removed from the market. Presumably, and hopefully, such actions were not arbitrary, but were the result of considered judgment that such deviation may be harmful to patients. Presumably, limits of ± 8 % on the labeled potency of digoxin tablets and ± 10 % for prednisone tablets (USP) reflect the conclusion that the dosage of these drugs should be reasonably well controlled and that a potency range of ± 50 %, for example, could lead to adverse effects.

We know now that two kinds of prednisone tablets might each contain the labeled amount of drug within ± 10 %, but that one may be completely, and the other only half absorbed, or not absorbed at all. We now know, in other words, that there is no necessary relationship between the dose given (other than in parenteral form) and the amount which is absorbed. This knowledge derives from our relatively recently developed ability to determine and interpret drug concentrations in biologic fluids, such as blood plasma and urine, and from our even more recent ability to quantitate at least some pharmacologic effects in man. With the application of these capabilities, it became apparent that we face bioavailability problems with many important drugs and that lack of bioavailability has caused, or has the potential of causing, considerable harm to patients.

I am often asked how many of our drug products are not adequately absorbed. Unlike epidemiologists who have numerator and denominator values to determine the incidence of a disease, we have no such quantitative information with respect to bioavailability problems, nor do we need it. When our colleagues, more than 100 years ago, set limits on impurities and degradation products in official preparations, they acted on the basis of their professional judgment that this was in the public interest, without arranging or waiting for a determination of incidence. If there were those among them who may have argued that the problem of drug contamination has been grossly exaggerated, and that the assessment of contamination was based solely on chemical assays with no one knowing really what constitutes a minimum degree of purity for therapeutic purposes, then history has mercifully chosen not to record their utterances and they, like the small number of our contemporaries who reacted similarly to bioavailability problems, have passed into oblivion. Our obligation is clear. We have to develop the means and set into motion those procedures which will assure that drug products not only contain the designated amount of active ingredient within established limits, but also that this ingredient is biologically available within defined limits. Setting one of these requirements without the other is irrational; any reasonably intelligent person would question our sanity if we insist on assuring tablet content within ± 10 % of label claim, while disregarding evidence that bioavailability can vary from 0 to 100 % as a function of pharmaceutical formulation. We must assure the bioavailability of our drug products to the best of our ability.

Relationship to Clinical Effectiveness

Bioavailability problems are, in essence, problems concerning clinical effectiveness. We know that there is a relationship between dose, or more exactly, drug concentration, and effect. This relationship may be relatively simple and easily identifiable, or complex and difficult to define. All other factors being constant, the intensity of drug action ordinarily increases with increasing doses in the therapeutic dose range. When a dose is not fully absorbed, its effect is decreased and the patient's condition may deteriorate. When a patient is treated with a drug product which is only partly absorbed, and he subsequently receives the same drug in a dosage form from which the drug is fully absorbed, then the effect of the drug will be greater than anticipated or desired, and serious adverse effects may occur. Clinical observations of both types have been made with anticoagulant, antiepileptic and anti-inflammatory drugs, among others. Because of the relationship between drug concentration in body fluids and therapeutic as well as adverse effects, the routine monitoring of drug concentrations in the plasma of patients is now advocated for many drugs.

Our own research efforts in the area of bioavailability led us some 10 years ago to initiate a program to determine the relationship between the dose or concentration of drugs in the body and the time course of drug action (1–4). Pharmacokinetic techniques are now at hand whereby rigorous correlations with pharmacologic effects can be made if good concentration and effect data are

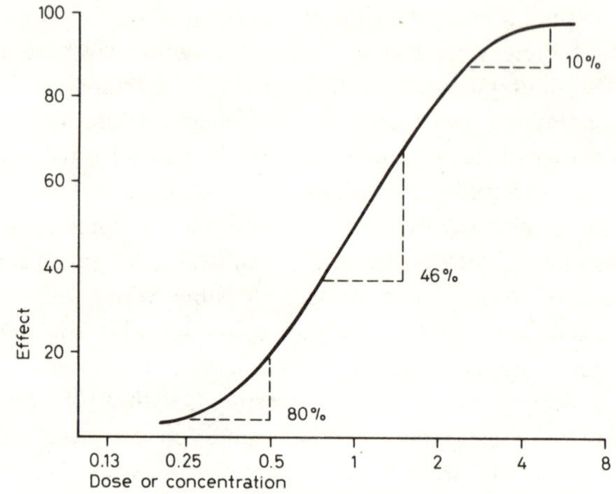

Fig. 1. Effect of 50 % decrease in bioavailability on pharmacologic effect.

available. For example, an effective quantitative characterization of the time course of the neuromuscular blocking effect of tubocurarine in man, as a function of dose and dosage regimen, has been accomplished (5). Even when it appears that there may not be any relationship between drug concentration and the clinically relevant effect, as in the case of the coumarin anticoagulants, such relationship can be demonstrated by the appropriate pharmacokinetic techniques (2). Apparent lack of correlation between drug concentration and effect, due to compartmentalization or activation phenomena, can also be rationalized and appropriate correlations can be developed (6). With our colleagues in clinical pharmacology focusing on the assessment of drug action and on the quantitation of pharmacologic effects, while we pharmaceutical scientists deal with the determination of drug concentrations in biologic fluids and the pharmacokinetic interpretations, it should soon be feasible to translate quantitatively the bioavailability data for many drugs into corresponding pharmacologic effect terms. Such translation is necessary because bioavailability and therapeutic effectiveness are related, but uniquely so for each individual drug and each drug effect. Let me illustrate this. The intensity of a pharmacologic effect is often linearly related to the *logarithm* of the amount of drug in the body in the central portion of the so-called dose-response curve. The entire curve is usually S-shaped (fig. 1). A constant fractional decrease in bioavailability will have a relatively much more pronounced effect on drug action if the dose is in the lower range of the dose-response curve. The usual therapeutic doses of most drugs are in the middle

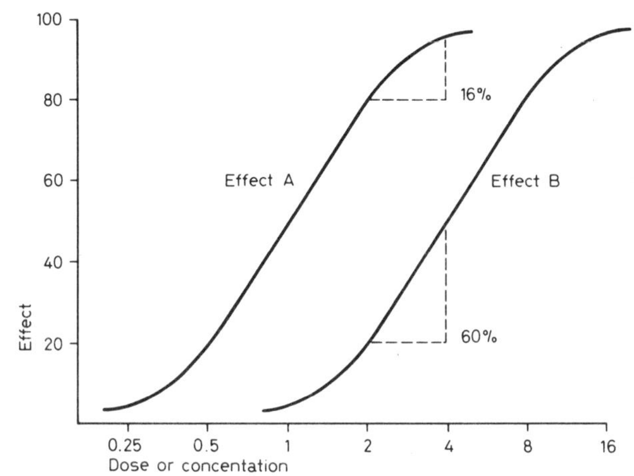

Fig. 2. Effect of 50 % decrease in bioavailability in two different pharmacological effects of a single drug.

or lower range of the curve and any decrease in bioavailability may decrease the drug effect more than proportionately. On the other hand, reduced bioavailability will not be reflected proportionately in the diminution of the effect of those drugs whose usual therapeutic dose is in the maximum effective dose range. The permissible bioavailability limits and the regulatory response to bioavailability problems should, whenever feasible, take this into consideration.

Most drugs elicit more than one type of effect, and it is often easier to quantitate one, rather than the other. Anticholinergic, diuretic, and neuromuscular blocking drugs are cases in point. The slopes of the different dose-response curves for a given drug are often (though not always) parallel (fig. 2). A decrease in bioavailability will affect each of these effects differently and it is therefore necessary to focus directly on the therapeutically relevant effect to assess quantitatively the clinical significance of a bioavailability problem.

The situation becomes somewhat more complicated in the case of drugs that are subject to dose-dependent elimination kinetics. Drug biotransformation and excretion were thought to proceed in man by apparent first-order kinetics, with the notable exception of ethanol. Some years ago we discovered, to our surprise, that the metabolic conversion of salicylate to its major metabolite salicylurate is easily saturated in man by administration of relatively small doses of aspirin. Since then we have found that several other drug biotransformation pathways in man, including certain sulfate and phenolic glucuronide formation and acetylation processes, are also of very low capacity (7, 8). As a consequence of this saturation effect, an increase in maintenance dose can cause a much more than proportional increase in the so-called steady-state or plateau level of the drug during repeated administration of constant doses at regular intervals (9). This effect is readily demonstrable and can be very pronounced; an increase in the daily maintenance dose of aspirin from 65 mg/kg to 100 mg/kg can increase plateau salicylate levels in the plasma 3-fold (10). Thus, an aspirin product with a bioavailability of only 65 % may elicit plasma salicylate concentrations which are only 33 % of those produced by a completely absorbed dosage form. When this is translated into anti-inflammatory effect terms, the difference is likely to be even greater because the appearance of certain adverse effects in the high dose range limits the therapeutic dose of salicylate to the lower range of the dose-response curve. That this is not speculation becomes evident from the clinical observation that an increase in dose of as little as 20 % can produce a dramatic therapeutic response in patients with rheumatic fever or acute arthritis (11). Also, our discovery some years ago that certain enteric-coated aspirin tablets were not fully absorbed was the result of observations by physicians that the particular products did not elicit the usual anti-inflammatory effect and pain relief in arthritic patients (12). Our pharmacokinetic data predict that such clinical assessment would, in fact, be feasible.

Any discussion of dosage-form effects on therapeutic efficacy cannot be concluded without emphasizing that incomplete bioavailability is not the only reason why the clinical efficacy of drugs may be impaired. Differences in absorption rate can affect the metabolic fate and the overall effectiveness of a drug even though the extent of bioavailability is not decreased (7). Adverse effects such as intestinal ulcers due to potassium chloride (13) and occult bleeding due to aspirin (14) are largely a function of pharmaceutical formulation.

The pharmaceutical formulation can profoundly affect the therapeutic efficacy of a drug even without changing the rate or extent of bioavailability. This is particularly shown very strikingly in the case of an aspirin preparation which contains sodium bicarbonate as a buffer. Even though the bioavailability of this preparation did not differ significantly from that of another which did not contain bicarbonate, the steady-state plasma salicylate levels were substantially different due to the change in urine pH produced by sodium bicarbonate (15). This effect is important only when high doses are used regularly, such as in arthritis and rheumatism; the smaller single doses used for the relief of minor pains are not as sensitive to the antacid.

These examples demonstrate the complexity of the decisions to be made and the different requirements for bioavailability testing, depending on the drug and its intended use. As I will emphasize again later in a different context, the biopharmaceutical assessment of drug products requires a comprehensive approach, with due consideration not only to the biomathematical, but also to the physiologic and clinical aspects of the problem.

The Public Interest

Having considered the need for bioavailability testing and the clinical significance of this problem, it is now necessary to establish what we should be doing in the public interest and in accordance with our responsibilities as scientists, health professionals, drug manufacturers, regulatory officials and legislators. We must accept the principle that the bioavailability of *all* systemically acting drug products, with certain obvious exceptions (such as intravenous injections) must be established and assured to the best of our ability. The time has come to undertake a review of the bioavailability status of all those marketed drugs which have not been assessed previously in this regard. The drug efficacy study undertaken by the National Academy of Sciences–National Research Council can serve as a model for such a project; the Academy of Pharmaceutical Sciences may be the appropriate body to carry out this task.

I am not so naive or uninformed to believe that bioavailability requirements can be instituted fully and enforced effectively in the very near future. There are technical, scientific, and manpower problems which have to be overcome. More about these later. What can be done, and what should be done now, is to adopt a policy of full disclosure whereby manufacturers are required to include an appropriate statement in their product literature if the bioavailability of their product has not been established. An analogous policy has already been instituted with respect to the clinical testing of drugs in infants, children, and pregnant women. The disclosure of the bioavailability status of a drug product will permit more rational drug and drug product selection for the benefit of the patient and will serve also as a powerful stimulus for the prompt acquisition of adequate bioavailability information where such information is at present not available.

There are specific aspects of bioavailability testing and decision making that require consideration: What is to be done if no chemical assay is available to determine the bioavailability of a new drug? What about the use of radioactively labeled drugs for bioavailability testing? Should the official compendia adopt standard formulas for dosage forms and should these be permitted to be marketed without bioavailability testing by each manufacturer? Should the innovator's product serve as the standard of reference for subsequently marketed products, even if it is not adequately absorbed? Are bioavailability studies in normal subjects adequate and appropriate for drugs used by patients with particular diseases? How can we find the medical manpower and human volunteers to carry out all necessary bioavailability studies?

Let me propose some answers to these questions.

It is conceivable that no adequate chemical assay is available to determine the bioavailability of a particular drug. Whether or not such a drug should be permitted to appear on the market becomes a matter of risk–benefit ratio. If the drug is truly unique and if its therapeutic index is such that some fluctuation in bioavailability is acceptable, or if its pharmacologic effect can be quantitated reasonably well so that it can serve as an acceptably precise bioassay, then it may be appropriate to permit the marketing of oral dosage forms without direct evidence of bioavailability. The point is that bioavailability requirements should never be applied out of context but as part of an over-all assessment of safety, effectiveness, and benefit–risk ratio. For the same reason, I consider it sometimes appropriate to utilize radioactively labeled drugs for bioavailability testing, despite the lack of specificity of the method and the problem of specially prepared dosage forms. If this method of assay is the only one available and the drug can contribute uniquely to the medical armamentarium, then the use of this method for bioavailability testing should be sanctioned. Very detailed and sophisticated *in vitro* dissolution rate determinations, to show that the tagged dosage form has the same release characteristics as the regular product, will have to be required.

In both of these special cases, further investigational effort directed toward the development of more suitable assay methods and the eventual assessment of bioavailability by standard procedures should be required as a condition for granting a new drug application. A precedent for this policy has already been established in principle with L-dopa.

It has been suggested that the official compendia or a group of small manufacturers might develop clinically-tested standard formulas for certain dosage forms, and that manufacturers who make these products need only be required to demonstrate that their products satisfy certain designated *in vitro* standards and tests. This proposal seems reasonable and attractive in principle, but experience suggests that it may be difficult to put into practice at least until very sophisticated *in vitro* test methods have been developed. Many pharmaceutical companies have been in the position of instituting the manufacture of some of their products in more than one location, often in more than one country. Despite identical formulas and manufacturing instructions, and often identical sources of supply of ingredients, there frequently occur pronounced differences between such nominally identical products. It is almost routine for some companies to send their production experts as trouble shooters to other manufacturing locations where they sometimes spend months to clear up such problems. Differences in batch size, humidity, quality of the water supply, competence of personnel, and other sometimes indefinable variables can account for differences in product quality. Very discriminating *in vitro* test methods may be required to determine subtle physicochemical differences which might have profound biopharmaceutic implications. Considerable time and effort will be required before it becomes feasible that such standard formulas do not need bioavailability testing by each manufacturer.

There have been instances where the innovator's product is not as completely absorbed as more recently developed competitive products. This is not too surprising, since the original product may have been formulated 20 years ago when the pharmaceutical sciences were not as well developed as they are today. Should such a product serve as the standard of reference and be matched in its absorption characteristics by the newly developed competitive products? I consider such a policy as bad science and as reflecting poor judgment. An incompletely absorbed drug is by definition variably absorbed. Depending on physiologic conditions such as gastrointestinal motility, its bioavailability can vary over a wide range. We have found that changes in gastrointestinal motility, due to thyroid disorders or resulting from administration of an anticholinergic agent, can change profoundly the extent of absorption of an incompletely absorbed substance in man. Drug products which are incompletely absorbed due to improper pharmaceutical formulation should be reformulated as soon as possible. Improved formulation and concomitant reduction of the amount of drug in the dosage form, to match the average blood levels produced by the original version of the product, are indicated. If newly-marketed competitive products produce higher blood levels than the innovator's product, then the latter should ordinarily be required to reformulate and all producers should reduce the amount of active ingredient appropriately so that the clinical effect of these products is in accord with physicians' expectations and previous experiences. If there be a common denominator for chemically equivalent products, let it be excellence and not mediocrity.

I have alluded already to possible effects of disease on bioavailability. There is evidence that not only thyroid disorders but achlorhydria, pyrexia, malabsorption syndromes, biliary atresia, and malignancy can affect drug absorption. Age, bed rest, and stress (such as that of blood sampling) are additional important variables. It becomes necessary, therefore, to consider the clinical indications and the conditions under which a drug product is used in determining the appropriate type of test subjects for bioavailability testing. I wish to propose a policy that is designed to serve these needs and that should increase considerably our capabilities for bioavailability testing, while at the same time enhancing the quality of medical care.

I propose that the bioavailability testing of generically equivalent drug products and the periodic re-testing of innovator's products be carried out in patients who require the drug for a sufficiently long time to permit determinations of so-called steady-state or plateau plasma or serum concentrations in crossover fashion. Such determinations of plateau concentrations are now being advocated widely to increase the effectiveness and minimize possible adverse effects of drugs (16). Bioavailability studies can be carried out effectively, with no additional expense, in conjunction with this kind of drug monitoring or clinical pharmacokinetics. Products would thereby be evaluated under realistic conditions, in the appropriate population, and without exposing normal subjects to unnecessary risk. The monitoring of drug levels is now becoming part of good patient care and thus constitutes a therapeutic rather than experimental procedure. Rapid analysis of blood samples combined with a policy of reverting to the previously used product if blood levels fall below a defined plateau will assure the patient of effective therapy at all times.

This type of bioavailability testing requires no additional medical facilities and is not dependent on a supply of normal volunteers. Comparative bioavailability assessments based on steady-state plasma levels have several advantages over single-dose studies: (a) the pharmacokinetics of drug elimination need not be known; (b) the assay need not be specific unless the patient also receives other drugs or certain unusual pharmacokinetic effects are operative; (c) single properly-timed blood samples on 2 or 3 days are sufficient, as opposed to the 10 or 12 successive samples required in single-dose studies, and (d) steady-state drug concentrations are often higher and, therefore, more readily measurable than those which can be achieved safely by single doses of a drug.

By instituting combined clinical pharmacokinetics and bioavailability testing programs, particularly in hospitals and extended-care facilities and in outpatient treatment centers, we will be able to improve the quality of health care for the general population because of the bioavailability testing program, and for the individual patient because regular monitoring of his drug levels in the blood will permit optimization of his dosage regimen and will help to reduce the incidence of adverse effects.

It has been only 10 years since the first comprehensive presentations of the scientific aspects of the bioavailability problem appeared in the medical and pharmaceutical literature (17–19). Much has been accomplished since then. A small group of dedicated and imaginative scientists has built the technical and scientific framework that can make the assurance of bioavailability a reality if government, industry, medicine, and pharmacy will commit themselves to this task vigorously and constructively. I have no doubt that this commitment will be forthcoming and that the quality of our drug products will continue to be a comfort for those among us who are ill and a source of pride for all who believe that this quality reflects the accomplishments of a free society and of people who care.

References

1 *Levy, G.:* Kinetics of pharmacologic effects. Clin. Pharmacol. Ther. *7:* 362 (1966).

2 *Nagashima, R.; O'Reilly, R.A., and Levy, G.:* Kinetics of pharmacologic effects in man. The anticoagulant action of warfarin. Clin. Pharmacol. Ther. *10:* 22 (1969).

3 *Gibaldi, M.; Levy, G., and Weintraub, H.:* Drug distribution and pharmacologic effects. Clin. Pharmacol. Ther. *12:* 734 (1971).

4 *Levy, G. and Gibaldi, M.:* Pharmacokinetics of drug action. Ann. Rev. Pharmacol. *12:* 85 (1972).

5 *Gibaldi, M.; Levy, G., and Hayton, W.L.:* Kinetics of tubocurarine elimination and neuromuscular blocking effect in man. Anesthesiology *36:* 213 (1972).
6 *Levy, G.; Gibaldi, M., and Jusko, W.J.:* Multicompartment pharmacokinetic models and pharmacologic effects. J. pharm. Sci. *58:* 422 (1969).
7 *Levy, G.:* Dose dependent effects in pharmacokinetics; in Importance of fundamental principles in drug evaluation, pp. 141–172 (Raven Press, New York 1968).
8 *Levy, G.:* Drug biotransformation interactions in man: nonnarcotic analgesics. Ann. N.Y. Acad. Sci. *179:* 32 (1971).
9 *Tsuchiya, T. and Levy, G.:* Relationship between dose and plateau levels of drugs eliminated by parallel first-order and capacity-limited kinetics. J. pharm. Sci. *61:* 541 (1972).
10 *Paulus, H.E.; Siegel, M.; Mongan, E.; Okun, R., and Calabro, J.J.:* Variations of serum concentrations and half-life of salicylate in patients with rheumatoid arthritis. Arthritis Rheum. *14:* 527 (1971).
11 *Calabro, J.J. and Marchesano, J.M.:* Fever associated with juvenile rheumatoid arthritis. New Engl. J. Med. *276:* 11 (1967).
12 *Levy, G. and Hollister, L.E.:* Failure of USP disintegration test to assess physiologic availability of enteric-coated tablets. N.Y. St. J. Med. *64:* 3002 (1964).
13 *Emerson, D.N.:* Potassium therapy and gastro-intestinal lesions. Rhode Isl. med. J. *53:* 378 (1970).
14 *Levy, G. and Leonards, J.R.:* The biopharmaceutics of aspirin-induced gastrointestinal blood loss. Farmaceutiskt Notisbl. *80:* 106 (1971).
15 *Levy, G. and Leonards, J.R.:* Urine pH and salicylate therapy. J. amer. med. Ass. *217:* 81 (1971).
16 *Vesell, E.S. and Passananti, G.T.:* Utility of clinical determinations of drug concentrations in biological fluids. Clin. Chem. *17:* 851 (1971).
17 *Levy, G.:* The therapeutic implications of brand interchange. Amer. J. Hosp. Pharmacy *17:* 756 (1960).
18 *Levy, G. and Nelson, E.:* Pharmaceutical formulation and therapeutic efficacy. J. amer. med. Ass. *177:* 689 (1961).
19 *Levy, G. and Nelson, E.:* USP and NF standards, FDA regulations and the quality of drugs. N.Y. St. J. Med. *61:* 23 (1961).

Author's address: Prof. *Gerhard Levy,* Department of Pharmaceutics, School of Pharmacy, State University of New York at Buffalo, 234 Health Sciences Building, *Buffalo, NY 14214* (USA)

Pharmacology *8:* 44–54 (1972)

Design of *in vivo* Studies of Bioavailability – Biometrical Considerations

J.E. Bearman[1] *and Ruth B. Loewenson*[2]

The Aspect of Definition

According to the flyer advertising the conference: 'Bioavailability of a drug substance in man relates to its appearance in the general circulation following administration in a pharmaceutical dosage form.'

Yet, prior to receiving the flyer, in checking with our friends in pharmacology, clinical pharmacology, and pharmacokinetics, we find that there might be several aspects to the problem: (a) dissolution and absorption (re: Dr. *Jollow*'s talk); (b) the rate at which the level rises in the blood; (c) the half-life in the blood; (d) b and c at the site of drug action, e.g. in the appropriate cells or in the inter-cellular fluids, and (e) urinary levels.

Thus, the very first problem for the very confused (and perhaps naive) biometrician is: Just which aspect of this elephant are we blind men examining? And in working with the clinical pharmacologist re: the biometric aspects of the design of studies in bioavailability, it may be true that in a single experiment we can study only one side, or at most just a few sides, of this many faceted problem.

A clear understanding of the problem at hand is a *sine qua non* for its solution. Perhaps most elementary science lessons have included some version of the following, which has become almost a cliché: more than half the solution of any problem is in its proper definition. And yet it may not be inappropriate to remind even as scientifically sophisticated an audience as this of such a simple principle. In just a moment in another context, reference will again be made to the importance of clear definition of the problem. While the aspect of definition of bioavailability may be of concern more generally, it is certainly one of the first interests of the biometrician in considering, what is for him, a new problem.

1 School of Public Health, University of Minnesota, Minneapolis.

2 Department of Neurology and School of Public Health, University of Minnesota, Minneapolis.

What Measurements to Make

Assuming we are able to decide on which of the various parameters we intend to study, we must then decide which measurements are appropriate. You gentlemen may feel this is no problem. But from bitter experience I can tell you that the simple matter of measuring 'blood sugar' had better be *carefully defined.* In a rather detailed protocol for a cooperative clinical trial, where it was clearly spelled out that 'blood-sugar' would be determined at stated intervals, by a method to determine true glucose values (not total reducing substances), it was early discovered to our intense embarrassment that, while most clinics were correctly using whole-blood, some clinics were using plasma and some were using serum.

For a naive biometrician this was hard to understand: the protocol clearly said 'blood-sugar'; blood is red, ergo 'whole-blood'. This was the intention; but some laboratories routinely use plasma for glucose determinations and that is what they used until we caught up with the misunderstanding.

Thus the measurements to be made must be explicitly defined so as to prevent misunderstandings – and then there will *still* be misunderstandings.

In this discussion I am assuming that the pharmacologists will be aware which measurements are relevant to the problem at hand, not just easy to make. Perhaps this is naive again, and perhaps this sentence should be included as this is one of the biometrical problems, viz. to be certain that the measurements are relevant.

Reliability and Validity of Measurements

Once it has been decided which measurements are to be made, and that these measurements are relevant to the problem at hand, then we must face the question of the *reliability* of the measurements. How well can an excellent technician, using aliquots of the same solution *but not aware that they are aliquots of the same solution,* how well do measurements on this same solution agree with each other? And how well do two technicians in the same lab, using aliquots of the same solution, agree with each other on the average? And how well will *different* labs, provided with aliquots of the same solution, agree with each other? There are some general answers to these questions, perhaps not very consoling: (a) There will *always* be variability in the determinations; (b) it is highly likely that there will be *less* variability of one technician with himself than between (and among) technicians, *even in the same lab,* and (c) there will be less variability within laboratories than among them.

So the problem is thoroughly difficult when we develop a method, and then propose its use on a general basis, across technicians (*not* all of equal excellence) and across laboratories.

Going along with this problem of reliability, or precision, is the companion problem of accuracy. Suppose we make up, with precise chemical methods, a solution to be sent to a technician or group of technicians, either in one or several laboratories. Now we know the exact quantity (per ml, for example) because that is the way the material was made up. And we may have previously assessed the reliability of the method being used (i.e. the variability in repeated determinations of the same solution). What, then, is the validity of the method in the hands of these people? How close to the true value will be the technician, or group of technicians, *on the average?* How accurate are the determinations on the average? To evaluate any method, we must determine both its validity and reliability over individuals and/or groups. These are both biometrically important aspects of the problem. The results of *Flokstra, Varley, and Hagans,* in the American Journal of Medical Sciences, vol. 251, pp. 646–655, 1966, diffuse rather interesting light on this problem.

The Appropriate Experimental Model

It is obvious, if we want results for use in humans, that animal models may provide excellent experience for preliminary work; but it must never be forgotten that animal work is just that: preliminary. While this is obvious, is it so obvious as to the kind of *persons* on whom we proceed to develop 'standard methods'? What are the ethical considerations of *developing* methodology using patients, who are ill? On the other hand, how relevant are data collected on normal, healthy subjects? Particularly if these healthy subjects are young, vigorous, but perhaps very overworked and fatigued medical students? How well does the absorption physiology of the target patient population compare with that of young, healthy students? Is there a difference in the uptake and rise of blood level between healthy subjects and those patients ultimately to be treated? How do the kidneys differ in their excretion rate and the liver in the breakdown and metabolism of the agents, so that conclusions can be drawn about the biological half-life in the patients to be treated? Of course, if preliminary information is gathered on healthy subjects, then it is possible (and necessary) to try out the agent on patients very carefully and to follow them closely, work them up completely and proceed slowly to the point where information on the target population becomes available. But where does one start and stop? These are not easy questions, and perhaps they are not strictly biometric in nature. But the biometrician must view very seriously these ethical problems, not only because they are an integral part of the problem, but also because he, too, must keep the ethical considerations always in view. In any case, if ever and whenever the subjects used in *in vivo* studies are patients, the type of subjects used must be *carefully* and *completely* characterized.

Interlude for Orientation

Perhaps it is time to come to the surface for a breath of air, and to try to orient ourselves. It is not unlikely that you may be wondering why a biometrician (or if you prefer to focus more sharply on me as a sub-specialist, then a biostatistician) feels the preceding topics are within his purview. If you expected something different, that too will come in due course. But there are at least two ways of performing *in vivo* studies, clinical studies, if the subjects are human. One of these involves clinical judgment and the global impression of the clinician. It might be fair to call such studies relatively subjective in nature. The other kind of study involves a definite attempt to simulate more nearly the conditions of a controlled laboratory experiment. Such a study might properly carry the description of being more objective in nature. While the subjective study may be perfectly satisfactory for some purposes, for example to convince the individual clinician of the efficacy of a treatment, there is little doubt that the subjective study is useless for other purposes. For example, for communicating the clinician's results to his professional colleagues, the subjective study has major shortcomings. It seems to us that our focus here is on studies that are to be communicable and communicated, so our aim is set on objective studies.

Objectivity depends on *all* aspects of data. These include proper study procedure and data collection; appropriate methods of recording the raw data, as well as the reduction of the data to tabular form, and proper analysis of the data as well as interpretation of the results. All questions surrounding the data are major concerns of the biostatistician. After all, his discipline is the one primarily concerned with data and its handling. It is for these reasons that I have imposed upon your time to remind you of facets which are, in our opinion, to be included in the *biometric* aspects of studies that you may perhaps think are not the business of the biometrician. The fact is that, if a study has a sound scientific logic in its basic concept, then the data coming out of that study should be analyzable, and usually by relatively well-known statistical models, even if not always simple models. If there is no known statistical model for a soundly conceived, scientifically logical study, then the biometrician had better get to work quickly and develop the appropriate methods for analyzing the study. That is his job. It is always possible, under the latter circumstances, that the methods developed may be beyond implementation. For example, it is not inconceivable that the proposed analysis might tax beyond its capabilities the largest computer available. Such was the case until relatively recently, certainly within the last 10 or 12 years, with some of the most innocent looking sets of data which had lost their orthogonality because of a small proportion of missing data. I am thinking particularly of a set of data that came to us concerning steroids, collected from newborn infants by one of our excellent pediatricians. The data involved 24-hour urine collections for a week, and it happened more than once that the catheter slipped out of a wriggling baby and went undetected for several hours or all night. Or some youngsters were discharged after 3 or 4 days, instead of remaining a full week. Other infants were not admitted until 1 or 2 days old, instead of being delivered on our OB service. Such events lead to problems in implementing an analysis, even though the *theory* might be completely worked out. Had such a set of data been presented to us in the middle or late 1950s, with the computers available then, instead of in the early or middle 1960s when a new generation of computers had been developed, the impossibly large load of simple arithmetic would have relegated the whole set of study data to the intellectual freezer until such time as the more powerful computers became available.

However, the other side of that same coin we have been contemplating is not even as sanguine as this. If the study is deficient in concept, and imperfect in scientific logic, then there is very little the biometrician can do to salvage the results with data manipulation. It is just as true with statistical formulae as it is with computers: garbage in, garbage out. And it is for this very cogent reason that I imposed on your patience to remind you of matters which, no doubt, are as apparent to you as they are to me.

Let me return, then, to those aspects of *in vivo* studies which you perhaps expect to be mentioned by a biometrician. The next group of four topics is related particularly to the collection of data. Biometricians are concerned with these matters because the proper implementation of these principles assures, as best as one can, that the data collected will be unbiased, the word 'unbiased' being used in its ordinary colloquial sense.

Placebos and Comparisons

The first of these principles concerns the use of placebos. Let me hasten to explain that I mean to cover more than what is ordinarily implied by that term. True, the meaning is 'a pharmacologically inert material, looking, tasting, smelling like the agent under test'. If there is *no* current standard agent in use for the same purpose as the agent under test, then it is satisfactory to use 'placebo' in its intended meaning. But if there is a standard agent, and the new agent is potentially a rival for that standard, or if we are testing a generic as a potential rival for a trade-name product, or vice-versa, then please understand my intent is *not* of 'placebo'; in this context, 'placebo' is correctly replaced by 'comparison-product'. The whole point is that *some* comparison is always necessary to demonstrate the efficacy of a product: does the product do better than nothing? Then a comparison group using placebo is a *sine qua non;* it is too late in the game to question the well-established fact that the placebo-effect is real and powerful over a surprising range of physiological as well as chemical parameters.

If the question is equivalence of one agent to another, or its superiority, then the advantages, really the *necessity,* of a concurrent comparison group hardly need to be mentioned.

Blind (or Double-Blind) Technique

How far need one go in emphasizing the second of this group of items, viz. the 'blind' (or even better 'double-blind') technique, where the subject (even better, both the subject *and* the clinician) is/are unaware of which agent the subject is given? It goes without saying that in a chemical or hematological laboratory determination, the personnel performing the test, count or assay must be 'blind' to which agent the subject was given. I hesitate to belabor the obvious to a group like this, and prefer to err on the side of omission rather than commission. Perhaps the only comment that need be made is that we must carefully avoid the 'triple-blind' situation wherein no one, including the statistician, knows what is going on!

Random Assignment of Subjects

It is equally true that, with a group such as this, one need not belabor the necessity for strict adherence to the random assignment of subject to agent. It will be recognized by all, that only with these randomization procedures are we justified in making the statistical probability statements we want to make in reporting our results. If one wishes to quote interval estimates of percentages of patients responding, or similar estimates of blood levels attained after a given time, and to state the confidence of such estimates, then the probability considerations surrounding such statements are justified only in the presence of such randomization procedures that have been used in the assignment of patients.

However, a word of caution must be mentioned. One must be certain of the *kind* of randomization one really desires. If global statements are intended to be made concerning the agent, over both sexes of all ages, and if patients are to be used over all severity categories, then one must be certain that the subjects in each group are *balanced* with respect to these variables singly and in cross-classifications. Such intentions can be implemented by a method of *restricted* randomization which, when properly carried out, assures the prior balance of the groups, yet introduces the randomization necessary for confidence interval estimation (or for p-value statements, which I find far less informative as well as far more difficult in being correctly understood by the non-expert). Where one wishes to draw conclusions about distinct groups of subjects, females separately from males, old in distinction to the young, etc., then we had best perform separate studies on the particular sub-groups of interest. This treatment of randomization is oversimplified and varies from situation to situation. In addition, it is an area replete with subtleties. It is difficult for me not to advise bringing in a statistically knowledgeable colleague as a member of the research team before proceeding with allocation of subjects to treatment. Perhaps I would be more myself if I were to recommend that a qualified biostatistician be a member of the research team at the earliest inception of any project and at all steps along the way.

Data Collection

It is necessary to say at least a word about the operational difficulties of data acquisition and recording. While it is well-disseminated doctrine in all areas of research that this data system must ensure uniformity and be comparable over time and space, etc., perhaps one point of very practical consideration concerns investigations involving humans: it is very easy to underestimate the work load. If one sets up to handle 3 new patients a week, there is little problem if these are one-time encounters. But if the investigation is designed for periodic repeat visits, it is not long before the traffic becomes jammed. From the point of view of the biometrician, the primary concern relates to the influence of expanded work-load on the quality of the data up and down the line. The immediate concern is that the pressure of numbers results in modification of procedures, non-uniformity in data collected, diminished precision in measurements and laboratory determinations and a general deterioration of the whole data system. In order to protect against such an eventuality, from whatever origin, the introduction of a meticulous system of quality control throughout the study operation can be the feature that ensures the success of a project. Warnings can be sounded and corrective action taken before serious damage is done, weak points in the system may be discovered early and strengthened, and breaches of protocol corrected before they become habitual. A good quality control program is well worth the effort and cost in its implementation.

Number of Subjects

Without doubt, what is expected of a statistically oriented person is for him to come up with the number of subjects needed. No one can do that bit of sleight-of-hand properly without understanding the specific problem in most of its details. For example, what size difference *makes* a difference; what is the magnitude, at least as a ball-park estimate, of the various known components of the variability, and of the experimental error; with what confidence are estimates to be made or at what significance levels do we plan to operate; what are the trade-offs in the risks and costs of the different erroneous conclusions that might occur?

From the impractical point of view, it is possible to determine the number of subjects with budget as no object, and reduce all errors to negligible proportions. Much more practically, it is possible to determine a whole spectrum of sample sizes, and the corresponding protection available in each case against the various kinds of errors and with various precisions of estimates. Alternatively, one can choose a sample size and, for given experimental error and patient variability, determine a network of available precisions and confidence levels; or if one is committed to testing hypotheses, one can determine a network of significance levels and minimal perceptible differences and the corresponding discriminating power of the test. These two latter alternatives appear most practical: budgets are usually real and limited, and a limited budget can provide a relatively fixed number of subjects. If the investigator can produce the necessary information concerning estimates of experimental error and inter-subject variability, and his needs concerning precision of estimates and confidence levels required, it is usually fairly straightforward to decide whether the limited budget can or cannot produce the kind of results desired. The very least that can result is that the whole project is judged too optimistic for the proposed budget, and the whole expense can be saved by not wasting it on a hopeless project. At best, the rational consideration of numbers required can lead to efficient allocation of limited resources.

Analysis of the Data

The one job recognized without question as the particular province of competence of the biostatistician resides in the area of data analysis. When we arrive at this stage of a study, we find that most of the previously considered topics focus on the problem at hand. Whether the results of the analysis will bear fruit that will be useful in advancing the whole project depends upon whether we have defined the correct aspect of the problem and decided on the appropriate and relevant measurements to be made. The validity and reliability of the measurements influence whether the results will be accurate and of sufficient precision in order to discriminate the required differences; the use of comparison groups and the double-blind procedure contribute to the same ends. Whether the appropriate experimental model has been selected is especially important as to whether the results obtained are applicable to the practical problem.

The random assignment of subjects directly influences the analysis. The specific randomization procedure is at the very heart of the statistical aspects of the design of the study; and the analysis of the data generated follows as a logical consequence of the design. That is, the manner in which the study was performed, its underlying logic, should inexorably determine the nature of the analysis of the data. It is for this reason that it is imperative that the biometrician have a complete and accurate picture of the entire study procedure in all its details. Without such information, it is too easy to have one's ideas misdirected as to the actual procedures that were carried out, and to proceed with an analysis of the data that does not truly reflect the conduct of the study.

For example, if a study is performed as a crossover design, i.e. each subject serves as his own control in alternating time intervals, then the analysis must reflect that design. If it does not, then incongruous findings may be the result. Similarly, a design that uses paired observations may be far better in scientific logic than independent samples; but if the fact that such a design was used is not made clear to the biostatistician, he may very well lose all the advantages of the more precisely conducted paired study by analyzing the results as if it had been performed as independently allocated samples. Conversely, to analyze a study with independent samples as if they had been paired-comparisons might very well erroneously ascribe a precision to the results that is not justified by the facts of the study procedure and the underlying logic of the study design.

These considerations bring us back to a point made earlier. If the biostatistician, as a member of the research team, is made aware of every detail of the study as it is performed, then he is in a position to plan the analysis of the resulting data as an accurate reflection of the study, and is also able to help maintain the performance of details of the study in conformance with the design. If he is not in such a fortunate position, then he is not able to help maintain the quality of data collection and recording, and he cannot be certain that his understanding of the total study is actually reflecting the conduct of the study in his analysis of the data handed to him. The use of a formula, or set of formulae, is not difficult; to understand the logic of a study, and to recognize the statistical model that correctly reflects that logic, is not a chore to be accomplished by some 'cook-book' process. Such a job requires a person to understand the problem, and who in addition has the talents and experience to translate that problem and its experimental setting into the appropriate pattern for analysis.

Interpretation of the Results

The interpretation of the analytical results, remaining within the framework of the mathematical model, be it a deterministic or stochastic model, should be an easy matter for the biometrician. However, to re-translate these results back into the practical, a biological setting may be another question. We revert again to the condition in which the biometrician finds himself.

If the biometrician is not fully familiar with all aspects of the study, as a knowledgeable member of the research team, he might do well to limit himself to the *formal* interpretation of the results. His interpretation of confidence interval estimates, or statements of statistical significance might best remain in the formal, probabilistic setting of the mathematical formulae. For him to go beyond this kind of interpretation might lead him into areas beyond his depth, where his interpretations (or misinterpretations) may be biological nonsense. In such a situation it is almost imperative that the pharmacologist-investigator be statistically knowledgeable.

Examples of this kind of misinterpretation of mathematics abound in the history of science. Even the great *K.F. Gauss* was misled in his work on the ether in relation to electromagnetic theory because he did not, apparently, understand the experimental results or else was not aware of them. In any case, he developed a purely mathematical formulation, not satisfactorily accounting for the observed experimental facts. At the same time, *James Clerk Maxwell* developed his mathematically beautiful equations, showing the reciprocal equivalence of the electrical and magnetic fields. Despite the fact that he had trouble accepting their implications, these equations accounted for all the known facts, and he was able to accomplish this outcome because he remained close to the experiments and let his mathematics be guided by the experimental results.

Such must be the case if the biometrician is to translate his results back into the field of application. He must stay close to, and be a part of, the studies; he must become a pharmacologist to more than a little extent if he wishes to help to translate his biometrical results into terms concerning bioavailability in man. And the more he makes himself knowledgeable concerning the clinical aspects of bioavailability, the farther he may safely venture to discuss the results of his quantitative calculations and their interpretation with his pharmacologist colleagues. But it must be emphasized that it is only the pharmacologist who is qualified to make the ultimate clinical interpretation.

Follow-up of Subjects

Finally, the aspect of the follow-up of the subjects who were in the studies is a dimension that must not be forgotten. This biometric component may be easily overlooked, and plans for this part of the study should be made early and carried out meticulously. Throughout the active phase of studies, provisions must be made for recording side-effects, and evaluating their occurrence in the treated group as well as in the comparison group. With complete information on the subjects over the short term, while they are in the active phase of the study, both numerators and denominators are available, and the comparative rates of occurrence of specific side-effects in the several groups can be evaluated.

However, it seems to us that the matter should not stop there in trials of human subjects. Untried agents may have unexpected side-effects which might show up at unsuspected intervals following termination of administration of the agent. Thus, it would seem prudent to plan on gathering follow-up data, at least on a minimal level for potential late-occurring side-effects, perhaps for as long as 3–6 months after termination of administration of the agent. Possibly longer or shorter intervals of such monitoring for side-effects can be planned with better understanding of the pharmacological fate of the drug in the human body. The point to be emphasized, from the biometric view, is that with this additional knowledge plans must still be laid beforehand in order to collect the appropriate data that will accomplish one of two things: (a) document the fact that the agent has no additional short- or long-term side-effects over its comparison agent, or (b) develop the data that it may have unexpected side-effects, over and above its comparison agent, in the shortest possible time using the fewest possible subjects.

Author's address: Dr. *Jacob Bearman,* University of Minnesota, School of Public Health, *Minneapolis, MN 55455* (USA)

Pharmacology 8: 55–101 (1972)

The Use of Physical and Animal Models to Assess Bioavailability

W.H. Barr

Department of Pharmaceutics, State University of New New York at Buffalo, N.Y.

The past decade has provided us with sample evidence that formulation variables can greatly affect the bioavailability and thus the clinical efficacy of many important therapeutic agents. Numerous *in vivo* and *in vitro* methods have been developed to assess these effects. We have not yet successfully applied them, however, to develop effective bioavailability standards in the case of many drugs for which standards are clearly required.

The recognition and correction of most problems usually follows the sequence: an initial recognition of the problem; accumulation of sufficient information pertinent to the problem; implementation of the information to effect a solution to the problem. Although there are still some who contend that there is no problem, it appears that we have passed the awareness phase. We are probably somewhere midway in accumulating necessary information and barely entering the implementation phase. To solve our present problem of developing products with optimal absorption characteristics and developing effective bioavailability standards will not be an easy job. It is my opinion that we will be preoccupied with this task for at least the next decade.

My assignment for this discussion is to review some types of physical and animal methodology which will be useful in our present implementation phase of developing effective standards to assure optimal bioavailability of marketed drug products. A comprehensive review of all potentially useful methodology would require several volumes of textbook proportions. In this discussion, I have attempted to give a few representative examples of the types of methodology which will be useful and some opinions on their relative merits and limitations when applied to various aspects of the multifaceted problem of optimizing and standardizing bioavailability of drug products.

Before attempting any discussion on the relative merits of experimental methods to assess bioavailability, one must first clearly identify the purpose for which these methods are to be used and the type of information that the methods might reasonably be expected to supply. The failure to recognize the distinction between these uses may result in disenchantment with a method potentially useful for one purpose because it was improperly applied to another; or may result in acceptance of a method for a use for which it is not the logical choice.

There are three major categories of information for which methodology is needed:

1. Methods to provide fundamental information on the physicochemical variables of the drug and dosage form and how these variables interact with the physiologic variables associated with the absorption process.
2. Relatively rapid, inexpensive and reproducible screening methods, which can be used in the development of new dosage forms to select candidates for further study in man or in the quality control of existing products as a secondary standard to detect potential deficiences in bioavailability which may indicate the need for further studies in man.
3. Direct methods to assess clinically significant differences in bioavailability which serve as the primary standard by which products are evaluated to determine acceptability for general clinical use.

Obviously, no single method will accomplish all these objectives. A method which is sufficiently sensitive and reproducible to quantitate small differences in the dissolution rates of several different salt forms of a drug may not be appropriate to determine the rate and extent of absorption of these forms in man.

It is well accepted that the ultimate criterion to determine the adequacy of the absorption characteristics of a drug from a particular dosage form is the clinical performance of the drug. However, the difficulty in quantitating effects in patients and the ethical implications of evaluating products in sick patients virtually eliminate this approach as a practical means for *routine* use. The method most useful in evaluating absorption characteristics is blood level studies in man, which allows direct quantitation and comparison of the rate and extent of systemic availability of the parent drug. The use of blood levels as the primary standard method is widely accepted by most authorities with the understanding that, for many drugs, our conception of the blood-level time profiles required for optimal clinical effect will undoubtedly change. The use of blood level studies and, in some cases, urinary excretion studies, in healthy volunteers will be the method of choice in most cases to set primary bioavailability standards. It is, however, conceivable that in some cases, new formulations may have to be tested in the patient population for which the drug is normally used if the disease process or other clinical variables alter the absorption requirements such that studies in normal subjects would not be predictive of clinically significant differences which would be observed in diseased patients.

The lack of sufficient human volunteers, the potential hazard in extensive human testing and the expense and time required, will obviously make it impossible to test every lot of every brand of a drug in humans. It will be necessary, therefore, to develop other methods which can serve as secondary standards to evaluate the bioavailability *potential* of dosage forms. The secondary standard should be a rapid, sensitive, reproducible procedure that does not involve human testing but has demonstrated correlation with *in vivo* bioavailability in man, which justifies its use in a predictive capacity to screen out dosage forms that are quite likely to show deficient bioavailability characteristics. It is axiomatic that as we move toward *in vitro* and animal methods, which may be more convenient, reproducible, or sensitive, we offset this gain by decreasing the probability that results of these methods will be directly correlated to the clinical effect. In very few instances will it be likely that the secondary method will be sufficiently predictive to obviate the need for testing in man.

The choice of procedures using humans, animals, or *in vitro* physical methods for basic studies or as standards to assess the bioavailability of finished products will depend on the relative weight given to the following considerations:

1. The sensitivity of the method to detect significant differences in the absorption characteristics of the dosage form relative to the clinical performance of the active ingredient of the dosage form.
2. The precision and reproducibility of the method in quantitating significant differences.
3. The relative safety of the method to patients and human experimental subjects.
4. The relative ease, time, and expense involved in the method.

Need for Fundamental Information on Absorption Mechanisms

The requirements of methods for research on basic mechanisms are quite different than those for routine use as a bioavailability standard procedure for quality control of finished dosage forms. It is the latter area that is of primary concern in our present deliberations. It is important to realize, however, that information on the basic mechanisms involved in the absorption of a drug is essential in developing new dosage forms and setting standards for existing ones.

In fact, without sufficient knowledge of the physiologic and physicochemical factors affecting the absorption of a particular drug, it will be difficult, if not impossible, to design procedures to routinely quantitate this event.

A schematic illustration of some of the potential rate-limiting steps in the absorption process and some methods to study them are shown in figure 1. The significance of each of these steps will depend on the drug being studied. For example, the release of drug from the dosage form into solution in the gastrointestinal fluids is often the rate-limiting step in determining the rate and extent of absorption. When this is true, *in vitro* measurements on disintegration, deaggregation, and dissolution, provide a rapid, sensitive, reproducible means to study these events that does not involve human experimentation.

For some drugs (e.g. aspirin) differences in *in vitro* dissolution rates of two products may be predictive of the differences in rate of absorption of the two products but may not reflect differences in the amount of drug absorbed. Differences in the rate of absorption may be clinically significant in some drugs which are used in single doses for relief of acute symptoms, such as pain or insomnia.

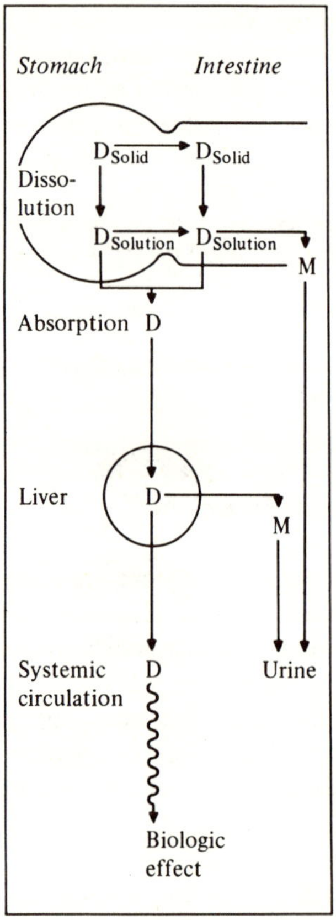

Events	*Methods*
Physico-chemical factors affecting drug release	*In vitro* physical methods direct measurement disintegration time dissolution rate
Membrane transport, intestinal metabolism, site of absorption, interaction between formulation variables and physiological variables	*In vitro* everted intestine *In situ* intestinal preps. perfused closed with sampling mesenteric v. cannulation
	Surgically manipulated unanesthetized animals
Hepatic metabolism during initial transit	
Systemic availability rate and extent	Blood level and urinary excretion in intact animals and man
Pharmacologic effect	Quantitation of pharmacologic effect
Clinical performance	Clinical studies

Fig. 1. Schematic illustration of some potential rate-limiting steps affecting the rate and extent of unmetabolized drug reaching the systemic circulation and methods used to study these events.

For other drugs (e.g. tetracycline) differences in dissolution rates may reflect a change in the amount of drug absorbed but not the rate of absorption because of differences in the rate-limiting steps involved in the absorption process. In this case, small changes in the rate of absorption are of no clinical significance anyway because they will not affect multiple dose plateau levels. These examples will be elaborated upon later in this discussion.

Frequently, differences in *in vitro* dissolution rates between drugs are not reflected in differences in blood levels in man. This may be because the *in vivo* dissolution step is not the critical event in absorption and attempts at *in vitro* correlation will be wasted effort. In other cases of poor *in vitro/in vivo* correlation, the method used may not adequately simulate the actual dissolution process in the human gastrointestinal tract.

For some substances, such very polar, water soluble drugs, e.g. quaternary hypotensives or vitamins, the rate of permeation across the intestinal barrier is the limiting step and information on *in vitro* (or *in vivo*) dissolution rates may be of little predictive value. The site of absorption in the gastrointestinal tract may be critical in designing or testing dosage forms of certain drugs. Although vitamin B_{12} is actively absorbed in the distal region of the small intestine, a formulation must permit dissolution in gastric fluids in order for the vitamin to combine with the intrinsic factor (secreted by the stomach) which is required for absorption.

It is now known that many drugs are metabolized by enzymes in the intestinal mucosal cell during passage into the mesenteric blood. Recent evidence shows that these intestinal and hepatic enzymes may be saturated depending on the rate and site of release of the drug, which greatly affects the systemic availability of the parent drug. Furthermore, it is possible that one drug of a multiple component dosage form may inhibit the metabolism of another, affect blood flow, or alter gastric emptying or intestinal transit.

To develop effective standards, it is necessary to have an understanding of the rate-limiting physiologic mechanisms involved in the absorption processes and how they relate to formulation variables. Judicious use of animal models and *in vitro* dissolution studies provide useful methods to elucidate these mechanisms.

Animal Models

Methods in Animals to Study Basic Mechanisms

To provide physiologically realistic experimental models without the expense and potential hazard of human experimentation, many *in vivo* and *in vitro* animal models have been developed.

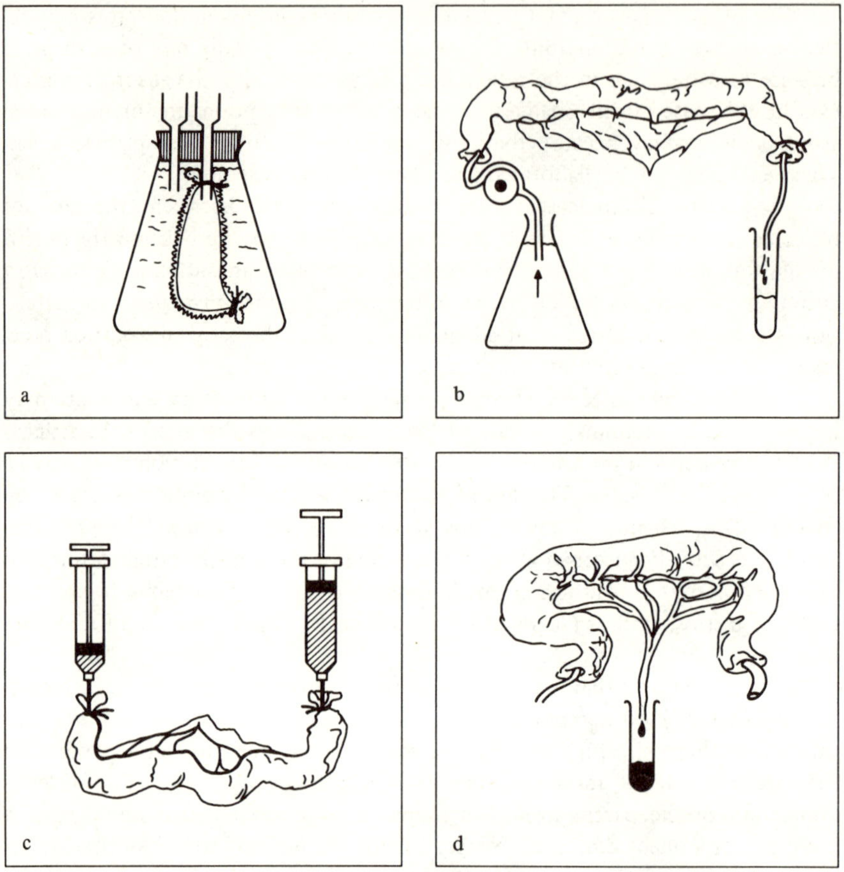

Fig. 2. In vitro and *in situ* animal preparations. (a) *In vitro* cannulated everted intestine; (b) perfused *in situ* intestinal preparation; (c) closed *in situ* intestinal preparation with intermittent sampling; (d) perfused or closed intestinal preparation with complete collection of mesenteric venous blood.

In vitro *Animal Models*

The cannulated *in vitro* everted intestine developed by *Crane and Wilson* (1) shown in figure 2a, is a simple and very rapid technique which has been used to study many factors which influence the transport of drug across the intestinal barrier, including active and passive transport, the presence of metabolizing enzymes in the gut wall, and the influence of other substances on membrane transport.

Several workers have used this technique to study active and passive transport processes (2–5).

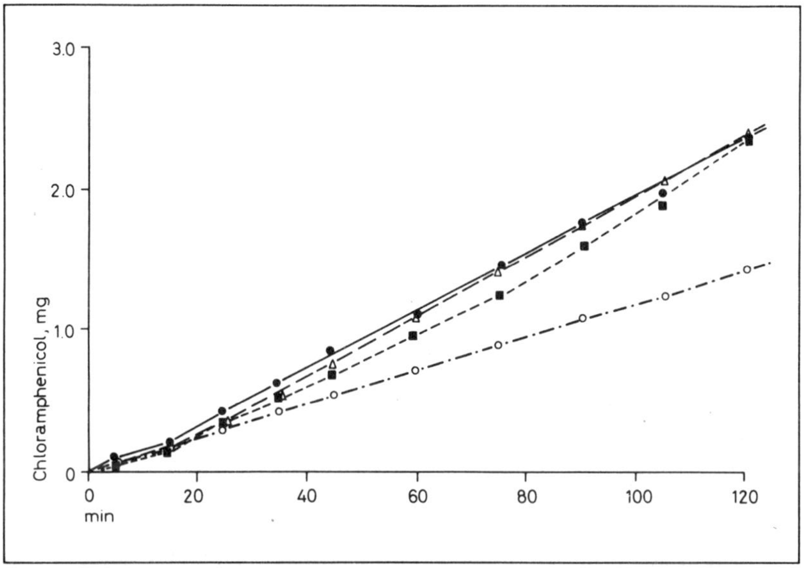

Fig. 3. Use of everted gut to study formulation variables. The influence of excipients in different brands of chloramphenicol capsules on permeation rates through the everted sac is shown. In the brand showing the lowest permeation rate (open circles), the excipients were found to coat the intestinal wall (3).

The everted intestine has been used to study the effects of various substances which can alter the transport of drugs by a variety of different mechanisms. An interesting application of this technique to study dosage form variables was made by *Aguiar* (6) showing that the excipients in one brand of chloramphenicol (fig. 3) capsules coated the gut wall and decreased permeation of the drug.

Reuning and Levy (7) have used this method to study the effects of complexing agents on drug absorption. Everted guts have been used by *Feldman and Gibaldi* (8) to study the effects of physiologic surfactants, and by *Saski* (9) for the effects of non-physiologic surfactants on drug transport.

Bennett et al. (10) and *Mayersohn and Gibaldi* (11) have shown that potassium and several electrolytes and sugars, such as glucose, decrease the transfer rate of salicylic acid and other drugs in the everted intestine. *Strahl* has found that glucose can either increase or decrease the permeation rate of salicylic acid and benzoic acid in the everted gut, depending on the concentration of glucose. Similar effects were not seen *in vivo* however (12).

The everted gut has been used to establish the existence of several drug metabolizing enzyme systems in the intestine which may play an important role in the absorption process. Intestinal enzyme processes which have been studied in this technique included aspirin hydrolysis (13), glycine conjugation of benzoic acid (14), salicylamide glucuronide and sulfate conjugation (15–17).

The relative rate and capacity of metabolite formation observed in the everted gut appears to correlate well with those seen in *in vivo* preparations (15) as shown in figure 4.

Inhibition of intestinal metabolism may be a consideration in some multiple component preparations which can be rapidly evaluated in the everted gut. The everted intestine has been used (17) to show that salicylic acid can inhibit the intestinal formation of salicylamide glucuronide by a competitive process and salicylamide sulfate by a non-competitive process increasing the transport of free drug over 50 %.

The everted intestinal preparation serves as the simplest method to rapidly examine *possible* effects of formulation additives on membrane transport and intestinal metabolism. Observed effects should then be confirmed by a more physiologically-realistic *in vivo* preparation with intact circulation.

In situ *Methods*

In situ methods have the significant advantage that although the animal has been surgically manipulated, the mesenteric blood flow is present, which obviates the non-physiologic transfer of drug across submucosal and muscularis barriers that occurs in *in vitro* methods.

Comparison of transfer rates in *in vitro* and *in vivo* preparations shows that the transfer rate of lipid soluble drug is much faster in *in vivo* preparations (15), not only because of decreased diffusion pathlength, but because blood flow creates a 'sink' condition. However, it has been reported that permeability of the intestine to large polar molecules increases in the *in vitro* preparations because of decreased cellular integrity due to hypoxia (18).

In situ methods can be classified according to whether measurements are made on disappearance of drug from the lumen or appearance in mesenteric blood.

The two methods which have been most widely used are the open perfused intestine (fig. 2b) and the closed loop methods (fig. 2c). The perfused intestine was used in the classic studies on the effect of pH on absorption by the Bethesda group (19, 20) and by other workers to study chemical structure-absorption relationships of sulfonamides and steroids (21, 22).

The closed loop method proposed by *Doluisio et al.* (23), which allows frequent sampling, is beginning to find wide use. Absorption rate constants obtained by this method appear to correlate much better with those obtained in the intact animal than rate constants obtained in the perfused intestine (23).

This technique appears to be an excellent approach for further studies on formulation factors affecting drug absorption. Recent studies using this method on a homologous series of alkanoic acids have provided an interesting extension to the pH-partition hypothesis and a better understanding of the relationships

4
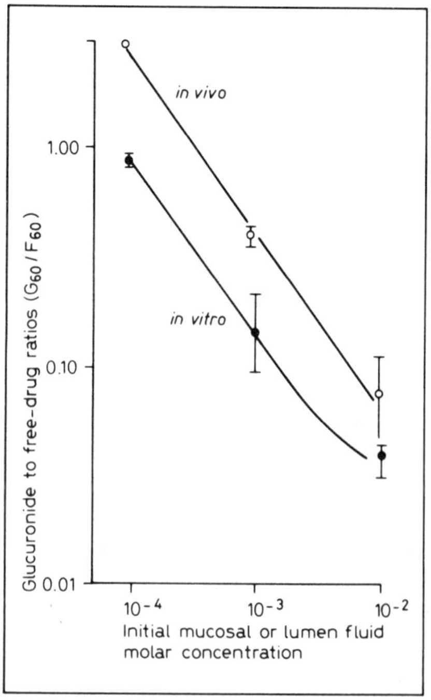

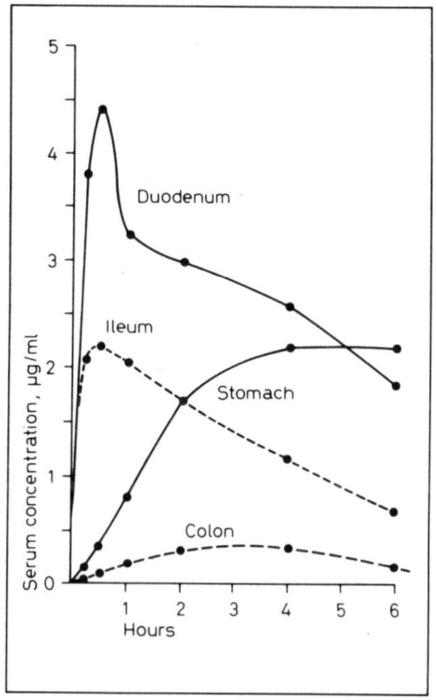

5

Fig. 4. Use of everted gut to study capacity of metabolic pathways. Comparison of the decreasing ratio of amount of glucuronide to free drug appearing in the serosal fluid of the *in vitro* everted gut and the mesenteric blood of the *in vivo* cannulated mesenteric vein preparation at 1 h as a function of increasing initial concentrations of salicylamide in the lumen fluid. Good correlation is observed between the *in vitro* and *in vivo* methods (16).

Fig. 5. Use of intact animals. Comparison of absorption of tetracycline from different regions of the dog gastrointestinal tract. The drug in solution was administered by cannulation into different regions (26).

between the physicochemical properties of the drugs and the rate-limiting steps of membrane transport (24).

One must exercise some caution with any method which measures only the rate of disappearance of drug from the lumen which may not equal the rate of appearance of drug in the mesenteric blood if significant binding, membrane storage or metabolism of the drug occurs in the tissue during transit. For example, it has been shown that disappearance of the same drug from the lumen was either mono-exponential or biphasic depending on the initial concentration used, suggesting two different absorption mechanisms. Observations on disappearance of drug from the lumen alone could not distinguish that this effect was due to saturable tissue metabolism (16).

The cannulated mesenteric vein preparation, in which all venous blood draining from a closed or perfused loop is collected, allows one to sample the mesenteric blood without the complications of the drug reaching the systemic circulation. Since all absorbed drug is collected in the venous outflow, the preparation can be treated as a closed system which facilitates kinetic analysis. This method has been used to study the kinetics of intestinal metabolism (16) and the effect of blood flow on free drug (15, 25) and metabolites (15). It has been used in dogs by *Pindall* (26) to study the *in vivo* dissolution and transfer characteristics of tetracycline.

Although this method is more difficult, it offers advantages for studies on drugs which are metabolized or stored in the gut wall. It can be used to validate the use of simpler methods which measure only disappearance of drug from the lumen.

Studies in Intact Animals

Small animals such as mice, rats, and guinea pigs, cannot be used to study intact dosage forms but have been widely used to study the relationships between the physicochemical variables of the parent drug (salt form, particle size, etc.), dissolution rates, and pharmacologic effects.

Excellent correlation between dissolution rates of various formulations and LD_{50} values have been shown for amphetamine (27), etryptamine, and benzphetamine (28), and a prodrug of acetaminophen (29).

The larger size and blood volume of the dog permits studies on intact dosage forms (capsules, tablets) using blood level measurements. Studies in the dog have provided early evidence of the effects of some formulation variables such as the pronounced differences in absorption of amorphous and crystalline forms of novobiocin (30). Blood level studies in dogs indicate differences in the bioavailability of salt, and free acid form of penicillin are observed when the drug is administered intragastrically but not when administered intraduodenally (31).

Harris and Riegelman (32) have used a surgically-prepared dog with chronically implanted cannulas to show the importance of the 'first pass' effect on the systemic availability of aspirin. Drug can be administered by cannulation techniques to various regions of the intestine. Betamethasone (33) and tetracycline (26) have both been studied in dogs by this technique as shown in figure 5.

Surgically prepared dogs with chronic gastric fistulas were used by *Lackman et al.* to study the release characteristics of enteric coated hydrochlorothiazide KCl tablets (34). Dogs with Thiry-vella chronic intestinal loops were used to study acetaminophen absorption (35).

Use of Larger Animals as a Secondary Standard

Use of larger animals, such as the dog, pig or monkey for routine testing of dosage forms, have obvious advantages relative to increased human safety and convenience in large crossover studies. They may provide a useful secondary standard for routine quality control of some drugs to indicate when human testing is required and may be useful in the development or screening of potential dosage forms.

For practical purposes the dog and 'miniature' pig are the most suitable candidates for use. The gastrointestinal physiology of the dog is similar to man with intermittent HCl and biliary secretion. *Poole* (36) has found reasonably good correlation between man and dog in absorption of dosage forms of penicillin derivatives. *Cressman* (37) has found that absorption of plain dosage forms of aminorex in dogs correlated well with results in humans, but that differences between sustained release preparations did not. *Rosen et al.* (38) found good correlation between man and dog in absorption characteristics of sustained and plain amphetamine products.

The miniature pig, which is really a small-growing animal, has found increasing favor as a research animal as it is comparable to man in many physiological functions. Being omnivorous, the pig's digestive tract is similar to man. There are two major limitations to use of the pig, however. Even though the size has been reduced, it still reaches about 200 lbs, presenting handling problems. Frequent venapunctures usually require a chronic cannulation. Secondly, the animal is continually growing, which may present problems in long-term crossover studies. The Canadian Federal Food and Drug Directorate is currently evaluating absorption in the pig using dosage forms of several drugs including phenylbutazone, sulfisoxazole and sulfadiazine (39). These studies, when compared to man, should provide useful information on the relative merits of studies in this animal.

It is perhaps too early to pass judgment on the use of dogs or pigs as a standard method, since there have been very few studies in which several dosage forms have been compared in both man and dog.

As discussed previously, it is important to distinguish between the use of animal models for basic studies and preliminary screening methods and their routine use as a standard for oral dosage forms intended for man. It is this reviewer's opinion that animal models are of great value in the first instance, but will be of limited usefulness in the latter.

There may be cases where data in these animals will be sufficiently predictive of results in humans to be used as a standard method. However, it is my opinion that at this point our time would be more profitably spent in developing better human models as the primary method and *in vitro* dissolution methods as the secondary standard. This conclusion is based on the following considerations:

1. Large animals are used in preference to an *in vitro* method in the belief that they will more closely simulate the human gastrointestinal tract. However, there are several differences in the gastrointestinal physiology of different species. These differences may offset the similarities. For example, *Weiner* (40)

has stated that tromexan is well absorbed in man but almost completely unabsorbed in the baboon.

2. Even if gastrointestinal physiology were exactly the same, differences in the disposition of the drug in the post-absorptive phase such as dose dependent metabolism, protein binding, renal or biliary excretion may greatly complicate comparison of blood level data in animals to that in humans. The fraction of drug metabolized by the intestine and liver during the first pass may differ greatly for different species. For example, dogs do not acetylate drugs. The extent of biliary drug excretion and enterohepatic cycling is frequently greater for dogs than man, which complicates analysis of absorption data.

3. Even when differences in products are detected in animals, testing in humans would usually be required before a dosage form is rejected. We do not know how often testing in animals would pass a drug which would not be acceptable on the basis of studies in humans.

4. The effort involved in dosing, collecting blood samples, and most important, the analytical work-up are essentially the same as required in human studies which will provide much greater information.

The use of animals in place of human volunteers rests on a decision whether an investigator is willing to introduce possible extraneous variables for reasons of expediency, convenience, or safety to human subjects.

We should recognize, however, that in the future, studies in animals may be required when the testing needs exceed the supply of human volunteers or in cases where the potential toxicity of the drug may preclude continued use in normal human volunteers, e.g. chloramphenicol or antineoplastic agents. We should, therefore, not rule out the possibility of using animals as standards for bioavailability. In this case, it must first be shown that studies in animals correlate with similar studies in man.

In vitro *Physical Methods*

In some cases the physical methods which will be useful in setting standards will involve direct measurement of a critical formulation variable, such as particle size (and distribution of particle size) or polymorphic form, which has been shown to correlate with decreased bioavailability. For example, an excellent linear correlation has been shown between peak blood levels of chloramphenicol and the percent of one polymorphic form of chloramphenicol in the dosage form determined by infrared spectroscopy (41). Direct measurements of particle size by various methods have been shown to have excellent correlation with *in vivo* bioavailability of spironolactone (42) and griseofulvin (43). Although the differences in these variables would also be detected by good dissolution methods, direct measurement is often a simpler and more reproducible means to quantitate differences in a specific formulation variable. In most cases, however, dissolution tests will also be required as the 'effective' particle size of primary particles in a finished dosage form and may also be dependent on manufacturing procedures (e.g. compression pressure) or excipients which determine deaggregation and 'effective' particle size. In some cases other formulation variables may be more important or may interact with the measured variable. For example, even though the particle size of a series of griseofulvin products were essentially the same, 3-fold differences in plasma concentrations were observed as a result of differences in excipients (44).

A complete discussion of physical *in vitro* methods should also include methods which characterize other events in the release characteristics of a dosage form such as release from hard capsules, tablet disintegration and deaggregation of drug particles, all of which have been shown to influence bioavailability. The reader is referred to other reviews which cover these topics (45–50).

Methods which quantitate specific formulation variables such as particle size or discrete events such as deaggregation will be useful in understanding the mechanisms involved and in some cases as a secondary standard. In most cases, however, the effect of formulation variables will be reflected by dissolution methods which measure the total interacting influences of formulation and manufacturing variables on release of active ingredient from the dosage form and will thus be the measurement most likely to be related to *in vivo* absorption.

A thorough review of even the methods that have been used to study dissolution would be quite extensive and is beyond the scope of this presentation. Fortunately, several excellent reviews are available including a recent series of comprehensive articles on the theory, methods, and *in vitro/in vivo* correlations by *Wagner* (45), a chapter by *Swarbrick* (46), and reviews by *Wood* (47), and others (48–50).

In vitro dissolution rate measurements have been used in a variety of ways including: (1) To study the effects of physicochemical variables of the pure drug on dissolution rates, e.g. salt, ester, polymorphic form, particle size, etc. (51–55). (2) To study variables such as manufacturing processes, tablet coating, excipients, on dissolution characteristics of the dosage form (56–61). (3) To screen potential dosage form candidates for *in vivo* bioavailability studies (62, 63). (4) As a retrospective study to explain clinical failures of a particular dosage form (64–67). (5) As a sensitive quality control procedure to detect changes in the release characteristics due to lot to lot variation, formulation changes, or storage conditions. These changes may or may not be detected in a less sensitive *in vivo* method (68, 69). (6) To provide an indication of differences in *in vivo* absorption characteristics of the drug and serve as a secondary standard to detect dosage forms with a potential for poor bioavailability (70, 71).

The use of *in vitro* dissolution methods as quality control procedures in the latter two functions have somewhat different requirements. When they are used

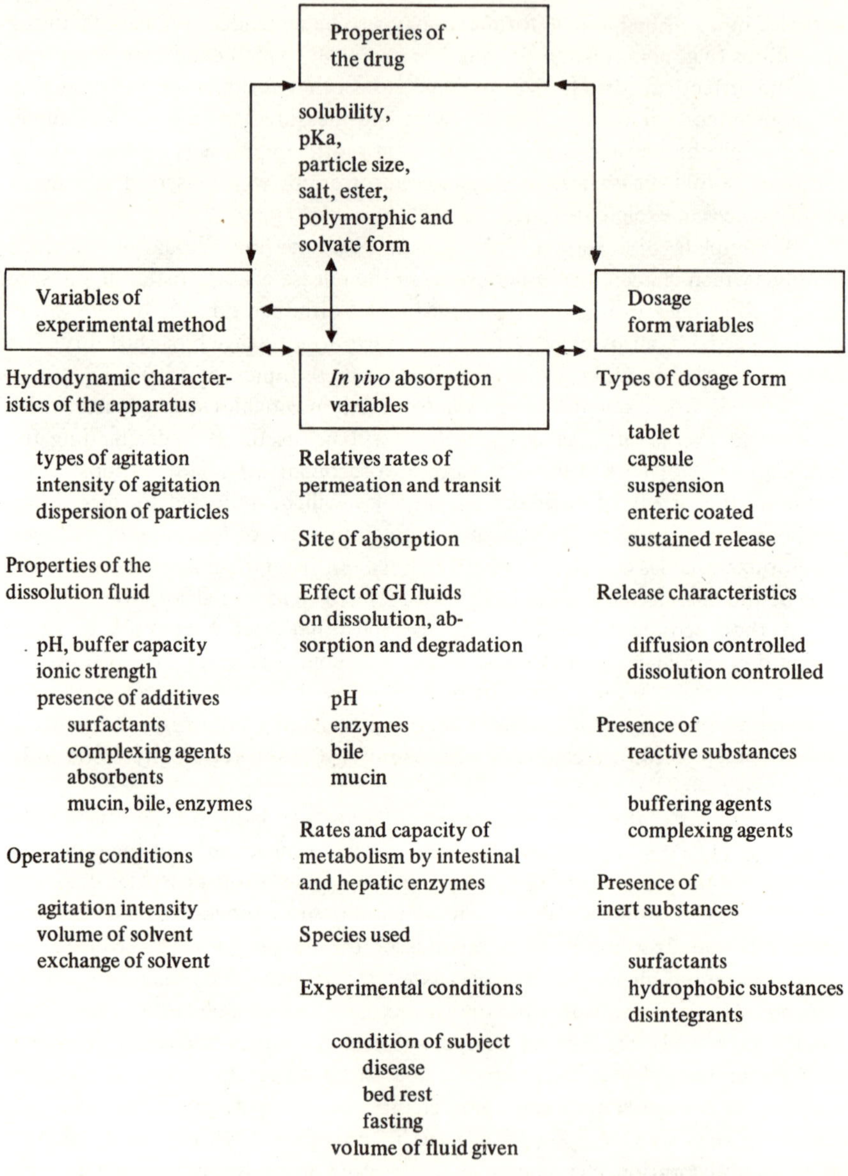

Fig. 6. Some interacting variables which influence the sensitivity and degree of *in vivo* correlation of *in vitro* methods to measure drug release and dissolution.

as a quality-control screening procedure to detect lot to lot differences or changes in the dissolution characteristics during storage of dosage forms, the principal requirement will be the sensitivity and reproducibility of the method to detect small differences. The differences may or may not be indicative of differences in *in vivo* bioavailability.

When they are used as a secondary standard to assess possible differences in bioavailability of products, the main requirement is a high degree of correlation between the *in vivo* and *in vitro* methods and the selectivity of the method to reject poor products but not acceptable ones. It will be much more difficult to find general methods that will be applicable to all products as a compendial standard to assure comparable performance of many different brands of drugs than a method that can be used by a particular manufacturer for his product alone.

There are thus two important characteristics of a given dissolution method – the sensitivity of the method to detect differences and the correlation of observed differences to those in *in vivo* bioavailability – either may be more important depending on the use.

The sensitivity and extent of correlation between *in vitro* dissolution methods and *in vivo* absorption parameters will depend on the complex interrelationships between the numerous variables of the drug and the dosage form, the mechanisms of absorption in the species tested, and the apparatus and experimental conditions of the *in vitro* method. A few of these variables are listed in figure 6.

Interrelationships between Mechanisms of Absorption and Correlation between *in vitro* Dissolution and *in vivo* Absorption

Knowledge of the relative magnitude of each of the potential rate-limiting steps in the absorptive process is essential in interpreting *in vivo* and *in vitro* studies and designing standards. The importance of this information will be illustrated by comparing three drugs: aspirin, tetracycline, and salicylamide. The contribution of each of the potential rate-limiting absorption processes shown in figure 1 varies greatly for these agents as shown schematically in figure 7 and further described below.

Aspirin

It is fortunate, albeit somewhat fortuitous, that so many of the early studies attempting to correlate *in vitro* dissolution with *in vivo* absorption were carried out with aspirin. Theoretical considerations on the relative rates of absorption and dissolution in both the stomach and intestine suggest that excellent correlation between the rates of gastric fluid dissolution and rates of absorption should

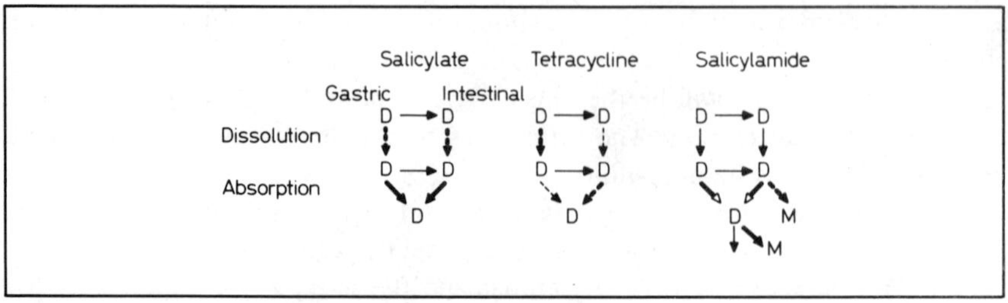

Fig. 7. Schematic illustration of the relative magnitude of rate-limiting events in absorption of salicylates (aspirin), tetracycline, and salicylamide. A large arrow indicates a relatively rapid rate. Small arrows indicate rate-limiting steps (see text).

be observed. This is true because of the following: (1) Aspirin in solution is rapidly and completely absorbed from both the stomach and intestine $t^1/_2 < 5$ min). (2) Absorption is rate limited by the rate of dissolution from the dosage form ($t^1/_2 = 15-100$ min). (3) Dissolution and absorption occur in both the stomach and intestine and gastric emptying is not a rate-limiting step.

8

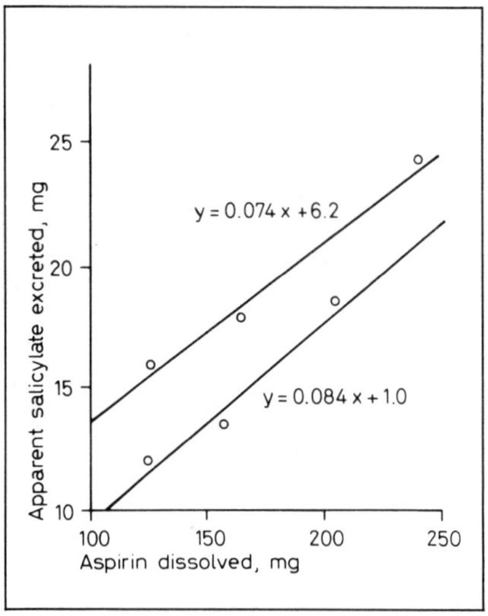

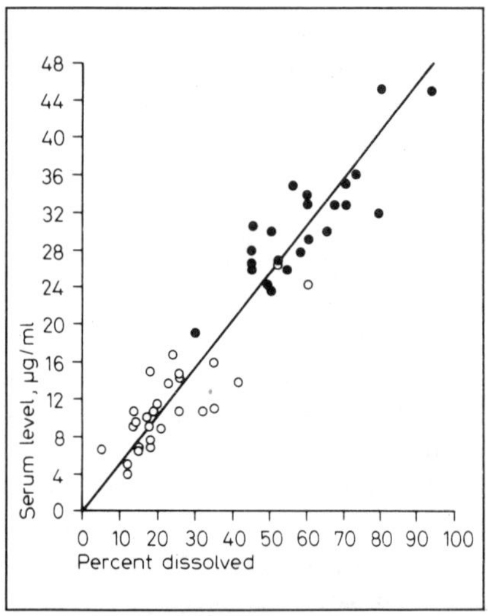

9

Fig. 8. Example of *in vivo/in vitro* single-point correlation. Correlation between total drug (as aspirin equivalents) excreted in urine 1 h after administration and amount dissolved *in vitro* in 10 min for three types of aspirin tablets. The two regression lines represent two different studies which differed only in the amount of water ingested by the subjects (100 or 200 ml) (100).

Fig. 9. Example of *in vivo/in vitro* two-point correlation. Correlation between 10-min serum level and percent dissolved at 1.2 min (○) and the 20-min serum level and percent dissolved at 4.2 min (●) (47).

It is not surprising then that excellent point to point linear correlation has been shown between the amount of aspirin dissolved *in vitro* in simulated gastric fluid and to the amount absorbed *in vivo.* These correlations have been shown for a variety of different types of formulations by *Levy et al., Wood et al.* and *Weintraub and Gibaldi,* shown in figures 8, 9, 10 and 11.

It should be noted that formulation factors usually affect only the rate of aspirin absorption and differences in *in vitro* dissolution rate will usually be indicative of only differences in the rate of absorption and not the total amount absorbed. The ideal properties of aspirin and the demonstrated *in vivo/in vitro* correlation with this drug make it an excellent model drug to further examine different factors which affect *in vivo/in vitro* correlations in the next section on relationships between dosage form variables and experimental variables in dissolution rate determination.

Tetracycline

The relative rates of the dissolution and absorption processes are much different for tetracycline than aspirin leading to almost opposite types of corre-

10.

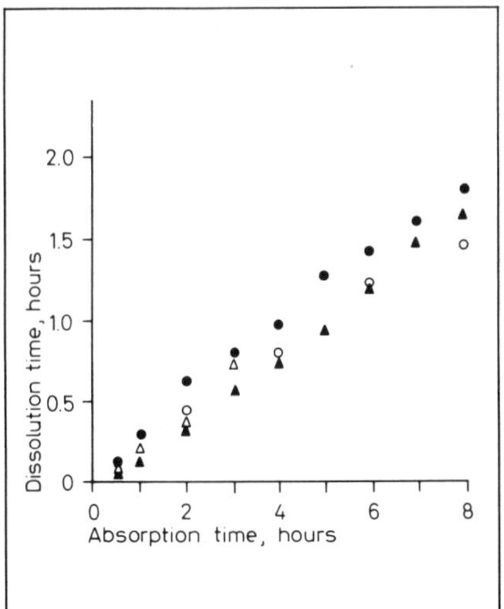

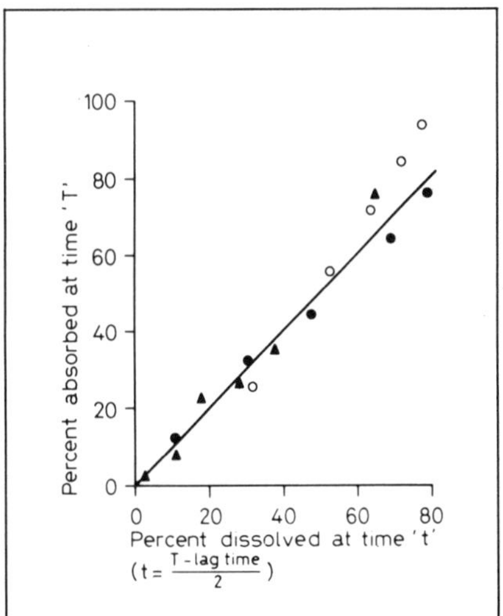

11

Fig. 10. Example of continuous *in vivo/in vitro* correlation (time). Correlation between the *time* required for a given amount to be absorbed and the *time* for the same amount to be dissolved *in vitro* for three sustained release aspirin products (47).

Fig. 11. Example of continuous *in vivo/in vitro* correlation (amount). Correlation between the *amount* absorbed at a given time (T) and the *amount* dissolved *in vitro* at time (t). The time, t, was selected to obtain a slope equal to unity. The abscissa time, t, is equal to the time for absorption T less the lag time, divided by the slope of a plot between the amount absorbed and the amount dissolved at time T (105).

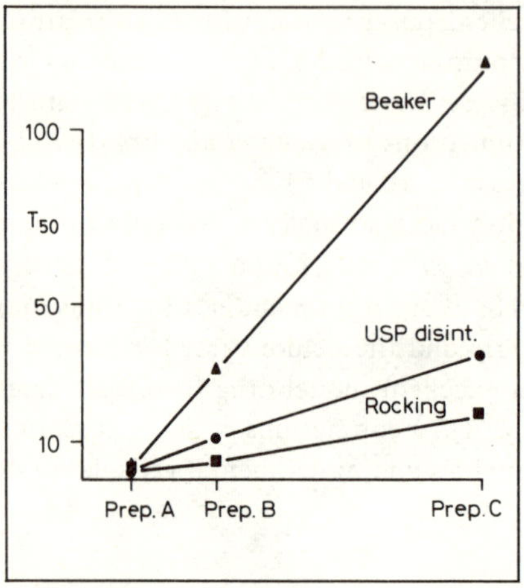

Fig. 12. The time required for 50 % dissolution (t_{50}) for three brands of tetracycline HCl capsules (A, B and C) in simulated gastric fluid in three types of dissolution apparatus, the *Levy* beaker method, the USP disintegration device and the *Lederle* rocking apparatus. The abscissa is an arbitrary scale to show the correlation between the three dissolution methods for the three products (72).

lations between *in vitro* and *in vivo* results. The mechanism proposed (72–74) for tetracycline absorption from solid dosage forms involves the following considerations. The solubility and rate of dissolution (72–74) in gastric fluid (pH 1) is much greater than in intestinal fluid (pH 5–7). Absorption of tetracycline in solution occurs much more rapidly in the intestine, however (26).

Drug particles which do not dissolve in the stomach are emptied into the intestine which is much less favorable for dissolution and generally will be unabsorbed.

The major rate-limiting step influencing the over-all rate of absorption ($t^1/_2$ = 40–60 min) is gastric emptying of the drug in solution. Thus, gastric dissolution rate will affect the *amount* absorbed but not the *rate* of absorption. An important consequence of this mechanism is that an attempt to correlate the amount dissolved *in vitro* at each time period with the amount absorbed *in vivo* at each time period, as was possible with aspirin, would be futile with tetracycline.

The rate of dissolution of tetracycline in gastric fluid should not be expected to correlate with the *rate* of absorption. Rather, the rate of absorption will be independent of dosage form, and differences in dissolution rate will correlate with only the amount of drug absorbed. Furthermore, one would expect that information on the rates of dissolution of tetracycline in intestinal fluids would also be required to characterize differences in the amount of tetracycline absorbed from different tetracycline products, particularly for those products which show poor dissolution characteristics in the stomach, in which case undissolved particles are likely to be emptied into the intestinal mileau.

Macdonald et al. found very good rank order correlation between dissolution t_{50} in simulated gastric fluid by the Lederle rocking cylinder and amount absorbed as determined by areas under the serum curve for 6 h and cumulative amount excreted in the urine in 8 h (75).

In our studies of three tetracycline products, we also found differences in bioavailability between products but essentially no differences in rates of absorption (76, 77). Dissolution t_{50} values in gastric fluid by three different methods showed excellent agreement between themselves as shown in figure 12. Although the sensitivity of the three methods is different, the ratio between $t^1/_2$ of the three products was remarkably consistent. This was also true for $t^1/_3$ and $t^2/_3$ values in the order $A > B > C$. If only sensitivity were important to distinguish between different formulations, then the beaker method is the most sensitive. It is possible that the rocking apparatus may provide a more physiologically realistic method with respect to agitation intensity and particle dispersion. The rank order did not correspond to actual bioavailability of the three products which was $A > B = C$ (fig. 13).

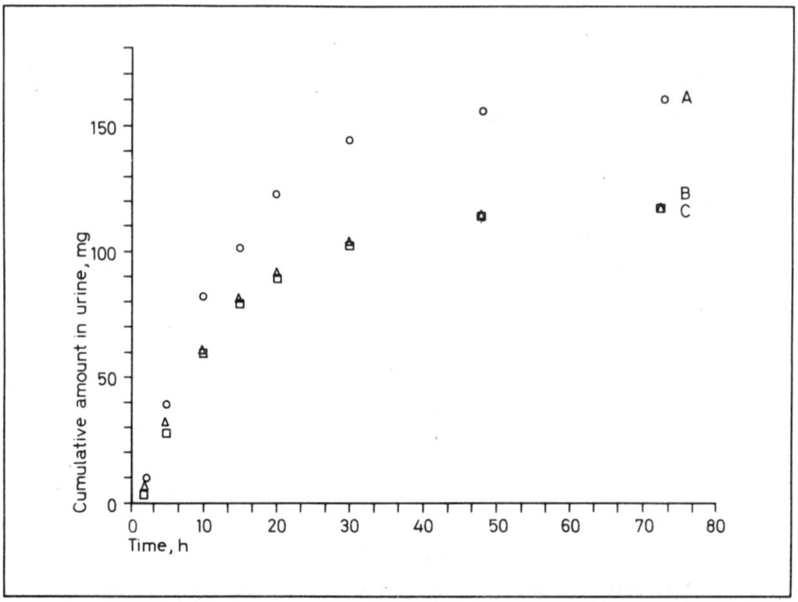

Fig. 13. Relative bioavailability of brands A, B and C as assessed by the cumulative amount of tetracycline excreted in the urine after 72 h (10 subjects) (77).

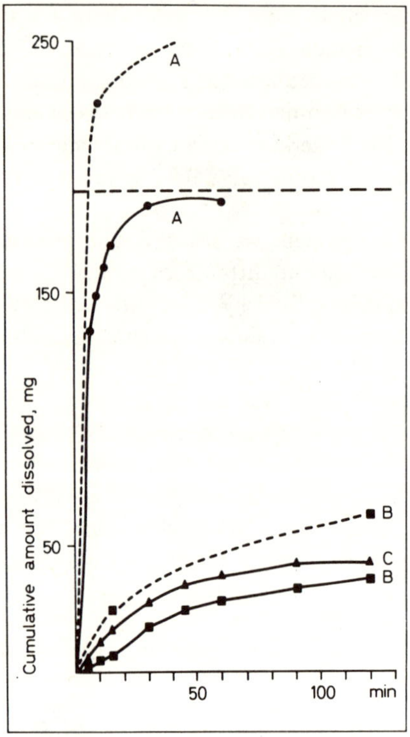

Fig. 14. Cumulative amount of tetracycline from brands A and B dissolved in simulated intestinal fluid in the USP disintegration device and the *Lederle* rocking apparatus (72).

The similar bioavailability of B to C is better understood when dissolution rates in intestinal fluids are compared (fig. 14) which shows that B and C both have similarly reduced dissolution characteristics compared to A.

The mechanism involved in the poor dissolution characteristics of brands B and C at higher pH values can be deduced by the dissolution behavior of the preparations in types of apparatus. In the USP disintegration apparatus, six capsules were studied simultaneously. The large amount of tetracycline HCl acts as a buffer to reduce the simulated intestinal fluid to a pH 5–6 which lowers the solubility by over 10-fold, a situation which may occur also in the intestinal fluids. Thus, in this method, the limiting factor of dissolution is solubility. When individual capsules of A and B were studied in the Lederle rocking apparatus, which has sufficient volume and higher pH to permit 'sink' conditions for dissolution, the asymptotic amount dissolved increases for brand A, but not appreciably for brand B in spite of differences in agitation and 'sink' conditions. It is probable that the poor deaggregation properties of B and C result in the coating of a tetracycline free base around the primary particle, which dissolves very slowly. Similar effects have been noted for warfarin (78) and benzphetamine pamoate (28).

A comment on the use of 'sink' conditions in dissolution methodology is warranted. It is usually assumed that for drugs which have a limited dissolution rate, the rapid removal of drug in solution by absorption creates a 'sink' condition *in vivo* (i.e. the concentration of drug in the fluids is less than 20 % of the saturation concentration). Therefore, it is desirable to design *in vitro* dissolution conditions to also maintain 'sink' conditions to insure good *in vivo/in vitro* correlation.

In the case of some drugs which are given in higher doses (250–1,000 mg) and are very insoluble (e.g. griseofulvin), or have poor membrane permeability characteristics (e.g. tetracycline), 'sink' conditions are not observed *in vivo*. This is clearly the case for griseofulvin. *Riegelman et al.* have shown that incomplete absorption of this drug from a solid dosage form continues for over 30 h (79). Thus, absorption of this drug appears to be solubility-limited rather than dissolution-rate limited. Examination of the literature and recent studies in our laboratory indicate that at higher doses (500–750 mg) tetracycline is less efficiently absorbed (i.e. dose dependent) probably due to limited solubility in the intestinal fluids (80). The degree of saturation of gastric or intestinal fluids immediately surrounding the particles will depend on the degree of dispersion of the drug particles as well as other formulation variables. It is possible that differences between products at saturation conditions may be under- or over-estimated by differences of initial dissolution rate in 'sink' conditions. Studies are not available at present on the correlation between dissolution rates in 'sink' and 'non-sink' conditions and *in vivo* absorption of dosage form of drugs in which *in vivo* 'sink' conditions are unlikely.

Effect of Bed Rest

Differences in *in vivo* agitation intensity and gastric pH during bed rest, an important clinical variable, may complicate the *in vivo/in vitro* correlation. The effects of bed rest on the cumulative amounts of tetracycline excreted in the urine following administration of two brands of tetracycline are shown in figure 15 (80). These effects of bed rest on the urinary excretion of tetracycline illustrate the complexities involved in assessments of bioavailability. It is difficult to evaluate the effect of sleep on absorption of a drug by blood level sampling for obvious reasons.

Thus, the use of urinary excretion of the drug has the advantage that the patient need not be awakened. However, although it is likely that the effects on decreased urinary excretion observed were due to differences in absorption as the effects were more often seen with brand B than brand A, we cannot rule out effects of bed rest on urinary excretion due to changes in splanchnic blood flow or renal function which might alter the relative fraction excreted in urine compared to the other major pathway of elimination – biliary excretion. Bed rest has been shown to affect the volume of distribution, fraction metabolized and excreted in the urine of several drugs including sulfonamides (81, 82), penicillins (83), and minocycline (84). These examples illustrate that we cannot make the assumption that either the absorption process or the subsequent disposition characteristics of a drug will be the same in normal ambulatory subjects as in sick bedridden patients. A complete understanding of these phenomena for tetracycline and other drugs requires further study.

Effects of Gastric Acidity

Further evidence for the importance of requiring adequate dissolution in intestinal fluid is given by a recent study (73) which shows that sodium bicarbonate, an antacid which does not chelate with tetracycline, decreases tetracycline absorption 50 % (fig. 16).

Patients with achlorhydria, gastric resections and other disease states resulting in high gastric pH may further augment the difference between products with poor intestinal dissolution characteristics. Furthermore, some studies indicate that the resting gastric pH may be close to neutrality. It is clear that optimally formulated tetracycline must have good deaggregation and dissolution characteristics in the full range of acidic and neutral pH values encountered in the gastrointestinal tract.

Dissolution Standards for Tetracycline

The important parameters for *in vivo/in vitro* correlation appears to be t_{50} values in gastric fluids which reflects the competing process of dissolution in the stomach and gastric emptying and the amount dissolved in simulated intestinal fluid preferably at the pH of minimum solubility (5.3) which is also within the pH of the duodenal contents and which reflects the dissolution and deaggregation characteristics of tetracycline particles emptied into the intestine.

Salicylamide

Salicylamide is essentially unionized at physiologic pH (pKa 8.2) and is absorbed extremely rapidly from solution from both the stomach and intestine.

Fig. 15. Effect of bed rest on the cumulative amount of tetracycline excreted when administered as capsules of brands A and B (80).

Fig. 16. Effect of sodium bicarbonate on tetracycline HCl absorption. Mean urinary excretion rates of subjects receiving a 250 mg tetracycline HCl capsule with 200 ml of water (•) or 200 ml of water containing 2 g of sodium bicarbonate (▲). Inset, semilog plots of urinary excretion rates in the postabsorptive phase showing similar 'half-lives' of elimination (73).

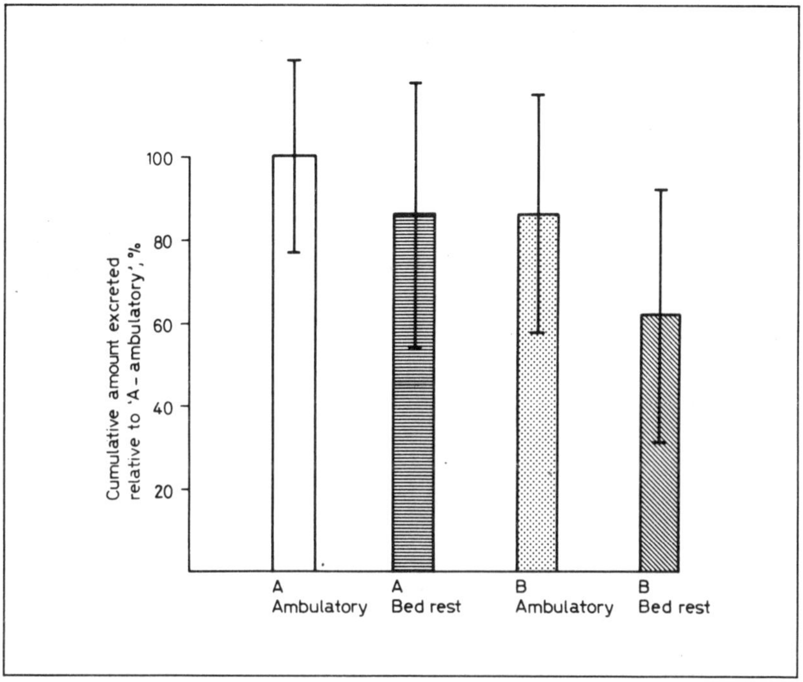

Cumulative amount excreted relative to 'A - ambulatory', %
100
80
60
40
20
A Ambulatory
A Bed rest
B Ambulatory
B Bed rest

15

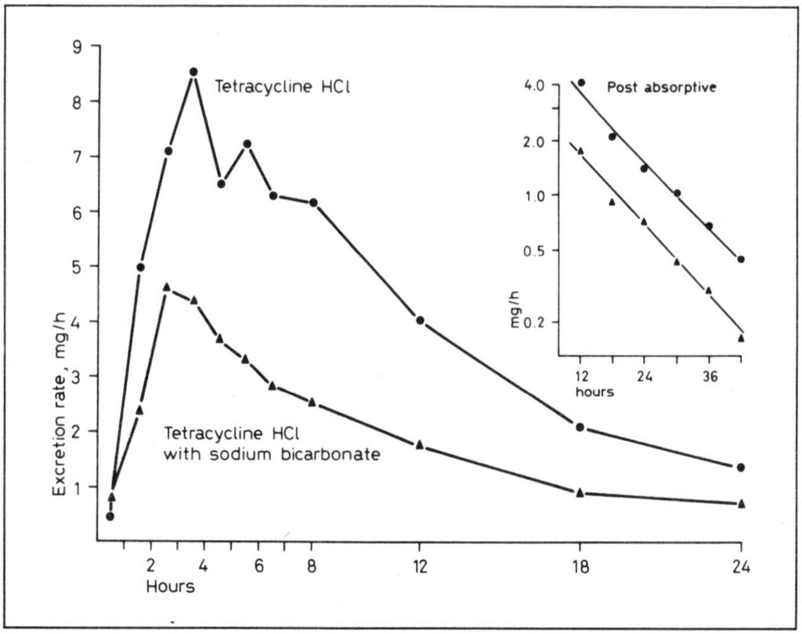

Tetracycline HCl
Tetracycline HCl with sodium bicarbonate
Excretion rate, mg/h
Hours
2
4
6
8
12
18
24
Post absorptive
4.0
2.0
1.0
0.5
0.2
mg/h
12
24
36
hours

16

At high doses, peak blood levels from solution have been observed within 5 min after ingestion (fig. 17). The drug is rather poorly soluble in both gastric fluids and intestinal fluids and is thus dissolution-rate limited in both regions. The feature that makes salicylamide an interesting model drug is that although absorption into the intestinal mucosa is dissolution-rate limited, the rate of systemic availability of free drug is metabolism-rate limited. Salicylamide is extensively metabolized by enzyme systems in the intestinal mucosal cell in the rabbit (15) and apparently also in man (85). It is also extensively metabolized by the liver during initial transit to the systemic circulation (first-pass effect). *Levy* has shown that changes in the dose and dosage form can change the ratio of amounts of salicylamide sulfate, and glucuronide appear in the urine (86) indicating saturable metabolism. Unfortunately, no free drug appears in the urine. Urinary excretion studies do not provide information on these changes in metabolism on the systemic availability of free (unmetabolized) drug. Studies on blood levels of free salicylamide (76, 85) following graded doses show that one or more of these enzyme systems can be saturated by a dose between 1 and 2 g of drug in solution. After saturation a small increase in dose (25 %) will result in 200–400-percent increases in peak plasma levels (fig. 17). However, when the drug is given in a dosage form, which slowly releases the drug, even doses greater than

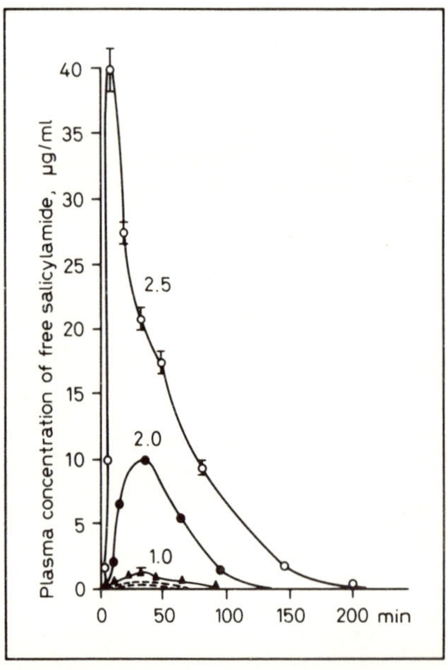

Fig. 17. Dose-dependent metabolism of salicylamide. Plasma concentration of salicylamide (free) following oral doses of 0.3, 0.5 (dotted lines), 1 (▲), 2 (●), 2.5 (○) g (85).

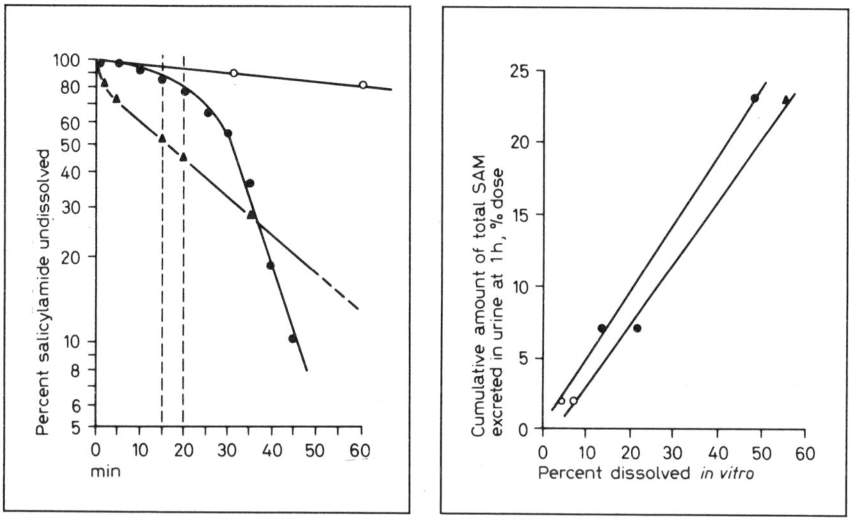

Fig. 18. Correlation of amount of salicylamide dissolved at 15 and 20 min and *total* drug (metabolites) excreted in urine at 1 h for a pellet (○), a commercial tablet (●) and commercial suspension (▲) (87).

1 g do not adequately saturate the metabolizing system, and blood levels of free drug may be quite small even though the drug is completely absorbed and appreciable metabolites are found in the plasma.

Unless the factor of dose-dependent metabolism during the absorptive phase and the lack of linearity between metabolite formed and free drug is recognized, unwarranted significance might be placed on apparent correlations between *in vitro* dissolution rates and total metabolites in plasma or urine. This may be true for example in the recent report (87) in which the amount of salicylamide dissolved in 15 and 20 min was found to correlate with amounts of total salicylamide (metabolites determined by acid hydrolysis) appearing in the urine at 1 h shown in figure 18. The choice of times was the same as that chosen by *Levy* in early studies on aspirin (fig. 8), but may be somewhat arbitrary as a crossover in the amounts dissolved between two of the products is seen at later times. This is incidental to the main point which is that any correlation with total metabolites of salicylamide, even though valid experimentally, may be misleading from a clinical point of view because total metabolites in plasma or urine give no indication of the pharmacologically active free drug.

This is clearly shown in figure 19 in which 300 mg was given i.v. and orally, resulting in the *maximum* differences that would be possible to obtain in both the rate and amount of systemic availability of free drug at this dosage level (a 100-fold difference). It can be seen, however, that total drug by acid hydrolysis

19 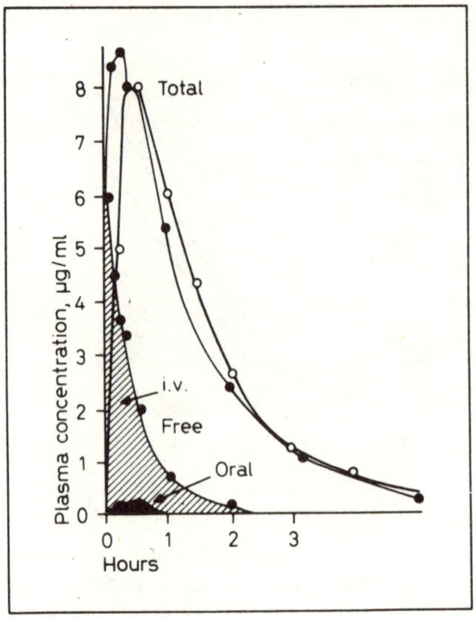

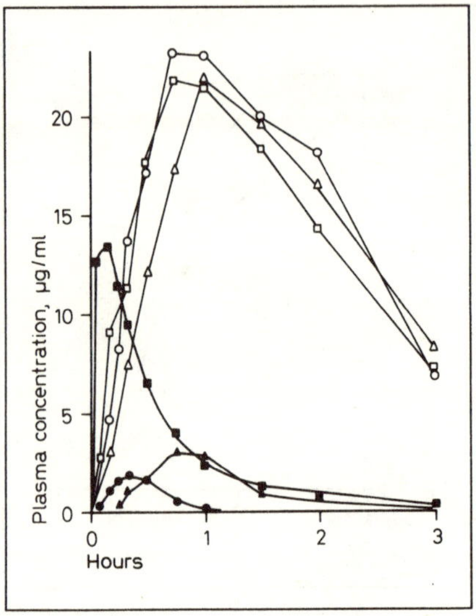 20

Fig. 19. Plasma concentrations of free salicylamide (shaded areas) and total metabolites (by acid hydrolysis) following 300 mg given i.v. or orally as a solution. Although great differences in free drug are observed, there is no significant differences in the plasma levels of total drug (85).

Fig. 20. Plasma concentrations of free salicylamide (closed symbols) and total metabolites (open symbols) following oral administration of 1.2 g of salicylamide as a solution (squares), a commercial tablet (triangles), and a commercial suspension (circles) (88).

is almost identical for both routes. At low doses (below 600 mg) very little free salicylamide reaches the systemic circulation because of extensive metabolism in the first pass. To be clinically effective, higher oral doses must be given so that enzyme systems will be saturated. When the same suspension used in the study cited above was compared to a solution and a commercial tablet at higher doses (1.2 g) there were large differences in the amount of free drug in the plasma but essentially no difference in the amount of metabolites in plasma (fig. 20) or urine could be observed (88). Furthermore, the dissolution rates of these products were not predictive of these differences (88). Most important, the suspension which appeared to have satisfactory bioavailability by measurements on total metabolite was found to have very poor systemic availability of free drug which correlates with the poor clinical performance of this dosage form observed in some clinical studies.

Thus, because of the absorption characteristics of salicylamide, *in vitro/in vivo* correlations using total drug are likely to be spurious, relative to the systemic availability of free drug. This example is not intended as either a criticism of the *results* obtained on the specific study cited above or others using total metabolite or total radioactivity since often this approach is valid (when the system is linear) or may be the only approach possible due to limitations in analytical methodology. It is intended simply to show that final interpretation of any experimental results is dependent on the amount of information on the mechanisms of absorption and disposition of the drug that is available at the time of evaluation.

Interrelationships between Dosage Form Variables and *in vitro* Dissolution Rate Methodology

Type of Apparatus

The most important variable in the sensitivity and *in vivo* correlation with *in vitro* dissolution-rate studies is the type and operating conditions of the apparatus used. The types of apparatus differ greatly in a number of respects including: (a) the type of agitation (e.g. laminar or turbulent); (b) the intensity of agitation; (c) the dispersion of the particles; (d) abrasion of the intact tablet or particles; (e) the volume and rate of exchange of the dissolving fluid relative to the solubility of the drug tested; (f) the flexibility of the system to vary volumes or agitation intensities; (g) the reproducibility of the system from run to run; (h) the reproducibility of the system in different laboratories which depends on availability of standardized components; (j) experience and documentation available for the method.

There are probably at least 100 or more different variants of types of apparatus that have been proposed. These have been reviewed in detail by others (45–50). Only a few basic types illustrated in figure 21, which have been extensively used or show particular advantages for studying dosage forms, will be briefly discussed relative to the criteria listed above.

Many early studies on mechanisms and formulation variables affecting dissolution rates of a drug, used static unstirred systems such as the hanging pellet method of *Nelson* (89) or the static disk method of *Levy* (90) in which non-disintegrating pellets or disks are suspended in solvent. These methods were used to correlate dissolution rates of salts of benzphetamine and etryptamine with median LD_{50} in mice (28), different salts and particle sizes of tetracycline with absorption in man (74) and different polymorphic forms of methyl prednisolone with implant absorption in mice (91).

Methods which have been used to study intact dosage forms have generally involved *induced* agitation by a variety of methods.

The most commonly used method and the one that should probably be used as a standard to compare others is the 'beaker method' used originally by *Levy and Hayes* (92). In this method agitation by stirring can be controlled. There have been several variations including the use of a round bottom flask by *Parrott*

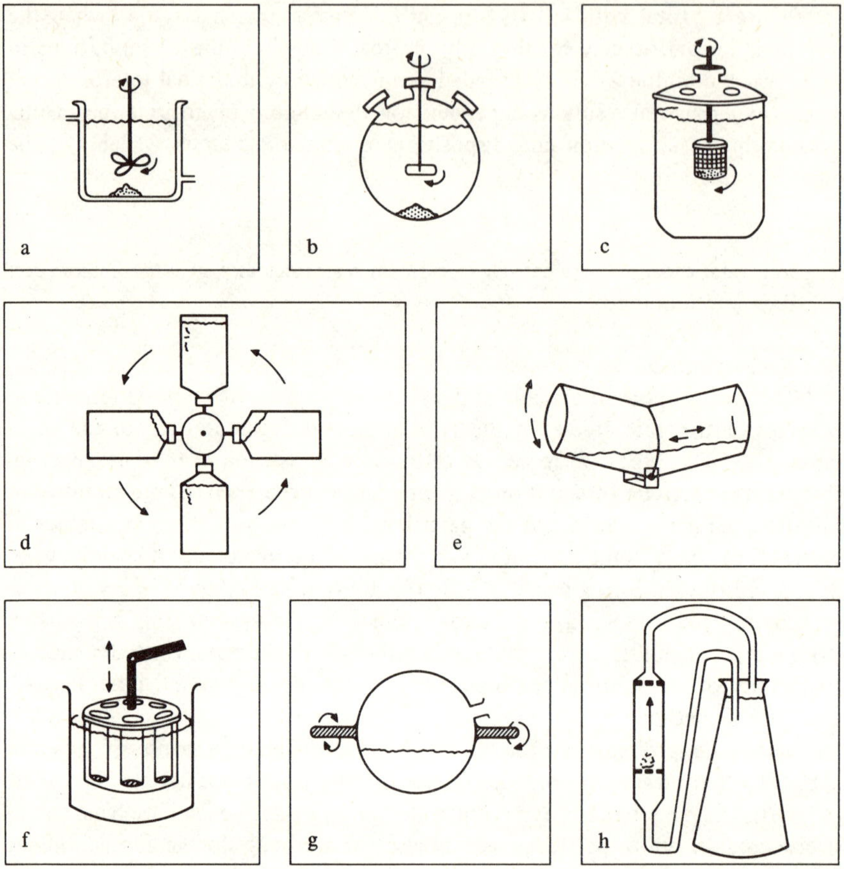

Fig. 21. Schematic illustration of some types of apparatus used for dissolution studies: (a) the *Levy-Hayes* beaker method; (b) round-bottom stirred flask; (c) the rotating basket; (d) the rotating bottle; (e) the *Lederle* oscillating or rocking cylinder; (f) the modified USP disintegration device or vertically oscillating cylinder; (g) the rotating round bottom flask, and (h) the flow-through cylinder.

(93), *Wood* (94), and *Poole* (36) with different types of stirrers. Changes in geometry of the container will affect the type of agitation (laminar versus turbulent) and the relative intensity of agitation as well as affecting the degree of 'mound' formation of particles on the bottom of the container due to poor dispersion of the particles.

The rotating basket method introduced by *Pernarowski* (95) and the current official method in the USP and NF is also subject to poor dispersion. The screen acts as an interfacial barrier at moderate stirring rates which is intensified by clogging of the fine mesh by undissolved particles. A further difficulty with this method is the abrasion of tablets produced by the fine (40 mesh) wire screen which decreases sensitivity. A combination of the beaker method with a basket fixed to the side is used by the FDD (96), which may also suffer from poor dispersion but probably has less abrasion of the dosage form than the rotating basket.

Weintraub and Gibaldi (97) have indicated that mound formation may affect apparent dissolution characteristics and that better *in vivo* correlations of some aspirin products was observed with the rotating flask which allows good dispersion at low agitation.

A similar type of dispersion is obtained with the horizontally oscillating or rocking tube used by the *Lederle* group (75) shown in figure 21. The rate of agitation is a gentle turbulent flow which is reproducible.

A modification of the USP tablet disintegration device (vertically oscillating tube) has been widely used because of availability and standardization and is currently official in the NF. It has a fairly high, inflexible, agitation intensity. The rotating bottle method originally developed for testing sustained release preparations is also difficult to standardize with respect to agitation intensity. When the bottles are rotated, the particles float downward at different rates depending on their density and shape.

The flow through apparatus of *Braun and Walker* (98) has shown good correlation with the *Levy* beaker for some drugs and has the advantage that agitation intensity can be precisely quantitated and mathematically described (99).

The significance of differences in the hydrodynamic characteristics of the different types of apparatus and operating conditions will depend greatly on the types of dosage forms studied. For reasons discussed previously, aspirin products serve as an excellent model to examine these factors.

Standard Aspirin Dosage Forms

Fortunately, many of the studies on aspirin have been done on the same three commercial dosage forms of aspirin which exemplify three basic types of formulations which have distinctly different dissolution characteristics.

The first is a 'plain' tablet which rapidly disintegrates into small primary particles. The dissolution rate is controlled by diffusion of drug from the saturated diffusion layer (microenvironment) immediately surrounding the effective surface area of the particles. The type and intensity of agitation can affect the dissolution rate by increasing dispersion of the particles and thus increasing the effective surface area and decreasing the thickness of the diffusion layer surrounding the particles.

The second dosage form is a tablet containing buffering agents (calcium carbonate and aluminum glycinate) in which the additives interact with the solvent and alter the pH of the 'microenvironment' immediately surrounding the particles. This preparation is very sensitive to additives in the dissolution media.

The type of third dosage form is a microencapsulated particle which is typical of many prolonged or sustained release products in which a nonreactive matrix surrounds the drug. The rate of release is dependent on diffusion of drug through the pores of the matrix. This type of preparation is relatively insensitive to changes in agitation intensity.

Effect of Agitation Intensity on Sensitivity to Detect Dissolution Differences in Aspirin Formulations

Many early dissolution procedures (such as the rotating bottle) were developed to assess the release characteristics of sustained release products. The relative success of these procedures, even though agitation was usually not carefully controlled, was because the rate-limiting step for release of drug from most sustained release products is diffusion through some inert matrix surrounding the dissolving particle. Even very large differences in the stirring rate (30 compared to 440 rpm) result in very small differences in dissolution rates from the slowly releasing microencapsulated particles as shown in the data of *Wood* in figure 22.

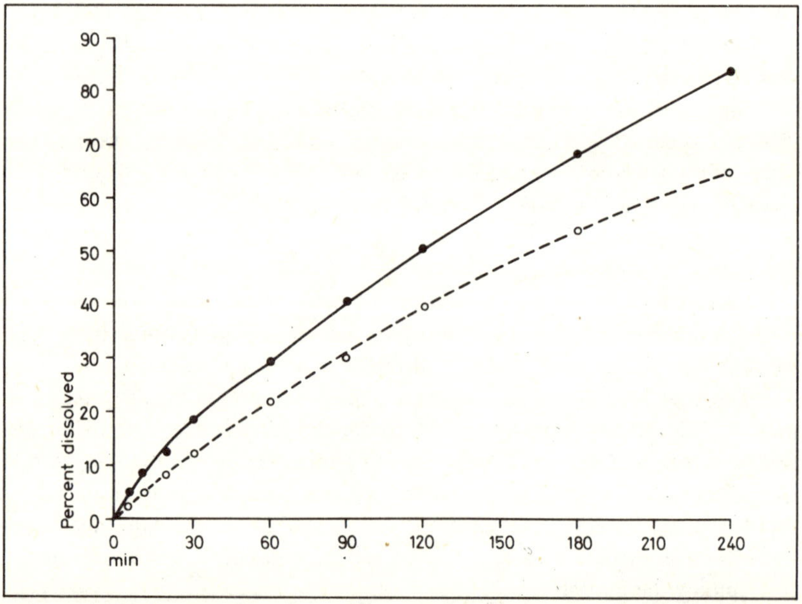

Fig. 22. Effect of different rates of agitation on the dissolution rate of a sustained release (matrix type) aspirin product. • = 30 rpm; ○ = 440 rpm (47).

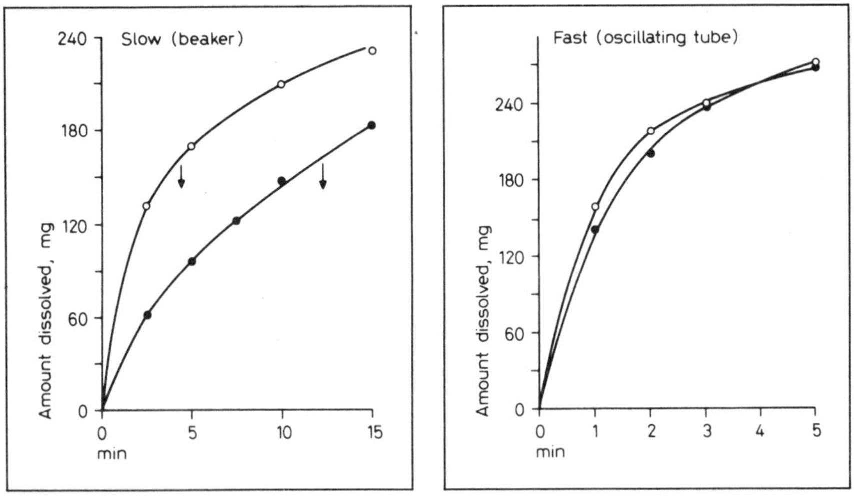

Fig. 23. Lack of discrimination between dissolution rates of plain (•) and buffered (○) aspirin tablets is seen at high stirring agitation intensities in the oscillating tube, compared to greater sensitivity of the low agitation intensity in the beaker method. Vertical arrows point to half-dissolution times (100).

Wood also found good correlation between the time for *in vivo* absorption and time for *in vitro* release in a round bottom standard flask (440 ml, pH 4 stirred at 420 rpm) for a series of experimental granules coated with ethyl and methyl cellulose (94). Similar correlation was obtained for three commercial sustained release preparations (47) (fig. 10). In both cases *in vitro* dissolution was about four times faster than *in vivo* absorption.

Wood states that stirring at high rates (ca. 400 rpm) could not distinguish between a 'plain' aspirin (A) and buffered aspirin (B) (47). Using much slower stirring rates in the beaker method containing 250 ml of 0.1 N HCl at 60 rpm, *Levy* found significant differences between A and B, which were not evident when the vertical oscillating tube method with much higher agitation was used (fig. 23) (100).

In both cases the high agitation rate produced by the different methods minimize the effect that the small amounts of buffering agent had on the microenvironment of the dissolving particles. It is interesting that while effects of reactive additives are minimized, the effects of some nonreactive additives may be more evident, at higher agitation intensities. *Levy* found that differences between products containing varying amounts of starch (5 and 10 %) were better observed by the higher agitation of vertical oscillating tube than the beaker method (fig. 24). *Wood* also found that differences between two products of varying starch content, which resulted in significant *in vivo* differences, were

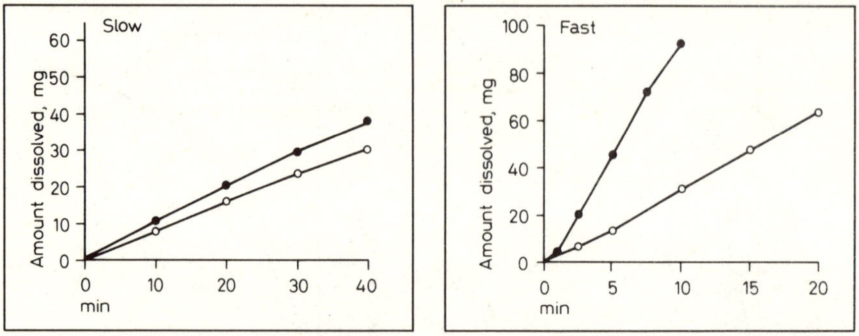

Fig. 24. Effect of agitation intensity in discriminating differences in dissolution rates between plain aspirin tablets due to a 'non-reactive' excipient (starch). As contrasted to the example in figure 21, better discrimination is observed between two products at higher agitation rate intensity (oscillating tube) than the slow agitation in the beaker. ○ = 5 % starch; ● = 10 % starch (56).

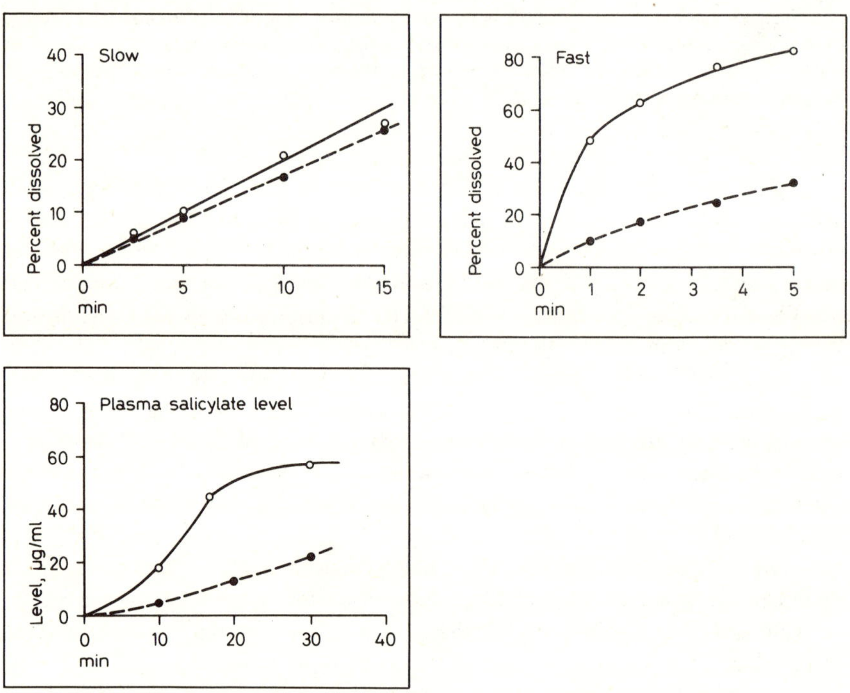

Fig. 25. Similar effects as in figure 24 in which slow agitation in the stirred round-bottom flask (ca. 30 rpm) failed to distinguish differences between two products of varying starch content which were discernible at high agitation (ca. 400 rpm). The bottom figure shows that these differences in dissolution rates are indeed significant relative to differences in *in vivo* absorption (47).

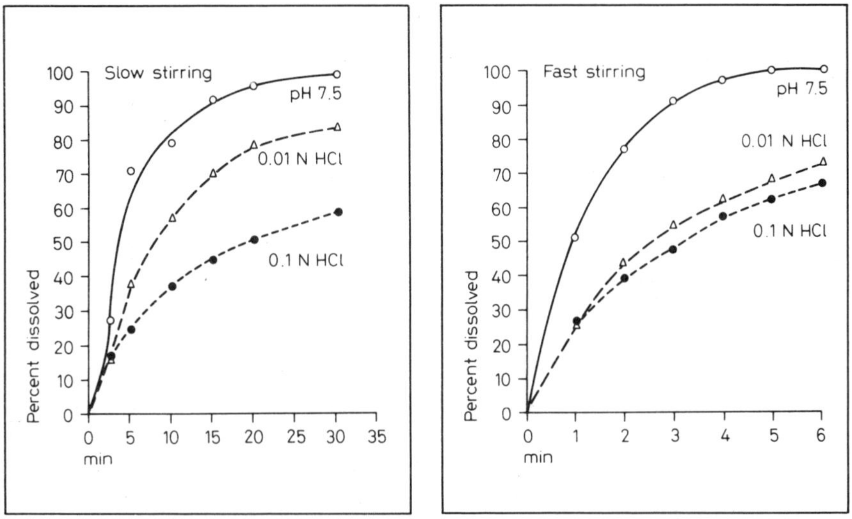

Fig. 26. Effect of dissolution medium on dissolution rate of Bufferin®. Interrelationships between solvent pH, agitation intensity and formulation variables. The differences between dissolution rates for buffered aspirin in 0.1 N HCl and 0.01 N HCl are masked by high agitation intensity (47).

evident at high agitation intensities (440 rpm) but hardly detectable at low stirring rates (30 rpm) in the stirred flask (fig. 25).

Kildig states that changes in dissolution rates of a product produced by storage was detected by the beaker method but not the round bottom flask (63), which may reflect the difference in 'effective agitation' intensities of these two methods.

Changes in Dissolution Media in Sensitivity

Changes in the pH of the dissolution media have the greatest effect on buffered tablets. *Levy* has shown that small changes in pH (about 1 pH unit) from 0.1 N HCl to 0.01 N HCl greatly increased dissolution rates of the buffered tablet, had only slight effects on a plain tablet and no effects on the timed release diffusion controlled preparation (101).

Further interrelationships between stirring rate, the pH of the solvent, and the effect of the buffering agents in the tablet on dissolution are seen in the data of *Wood* in figure 26. At low stirring rates (30 rpm) the rate of dissolution in 0.01 N HCl is significantly different between the plain and buffered tablet. These differences are minimized when agitation is increased to 440 rpm.

A different effect of additives on dissolution of the buffered tablet was suggested by *Levy* to explain the pronounced increase in dissolution rate of the buffered tablet when citric acid is added to the dissolving medium. Addition of citric acid has virtually no effect on the plain tablet or microencapsulated sustained release product. *Levy* suggests that citric acid complexes with the aluminum component of the buffer to prevent build-up of insoluble aluminum salts (101).

Weintraub and Gibaldi found that addition of a surfactant (0.01 % Brij 35SP) increased the dissolution rate of the buffered tablet in the stirred round bottom flask presumably because of increased wetting of the porous mound but decreased the dissolution rate of the buffered tablet in the rotating flask where dispersion is more efficient and a 'mound' does not occur (97, 102).

Choice of Agitation Intensity to Optimize in vivo/in vitro *Correlation*

The series of excellent studies of *Levy et al.* during the past 10 years have provided considerable insight into the complexities involved in calibrating *in vitro* agitation intensity with *in vivo* absorption. *Levy* first used the data of *Leonards* and the method of *Wagner and Nelson* to determine the amount of aspirin absorbed (as salicylic acid) from plain and buffered aspirin tablets as a function of time (103). An excellent linear correlation was shown by both plain and buffered aspirin between the amount dissolved at a given time in the beaker method (250 ml, 1 N HCl, 60 rpm) and the amount absorbed (fig. 27). It is seen in this plot that an intercept exists which is presumably due to the lag time for absorption *in vivo*. The linear regression with a slope of 3 occurs until about 80 % is dissolved. That is, the *in vitro* dissolution is consistently three times as fast as the *in vivo* absorption. This ratio is referred to as the intensity factor. In this case the intensity factor is determined by both the *in vivo/in vitro* conditions which were somewhat arbitrary. The factor would have been different, for example, if slightly different agitation intensities were used. Two subsequent studies by *Levy et al.* illustrate this point.

In the second separate study, *Levy and Hollister* gave three tablets (975 mg) of aspirin (a different brand than previously used) to ten subjects and again correlated the amount absorbed at a given time with the amount dissolved in a procedure somewhat different from the first study. A larger volume (350 ml) was used and data in which the dissolving tablet formed a mound on the side rather than the center of the beaker was excluded (104).

The *in vivo/in vitro* linear correlation obtained (fig. 28) is as good as the previous study but the intensity factor or ratio between *in vivo* and *in vitro* rates was 8.5, almost three times that previously obtained. It is not possible to establish the reason for this increase. There are probably several contributing factors. The *in vitro* dissolution rates were increased by increasing the volume (increasing 'sink' conditions) and omitting data where mound formation occurred on the side of the beaker. *Swarbrick* (46) has shown that the rates of dissolution in these two instances are quite different.

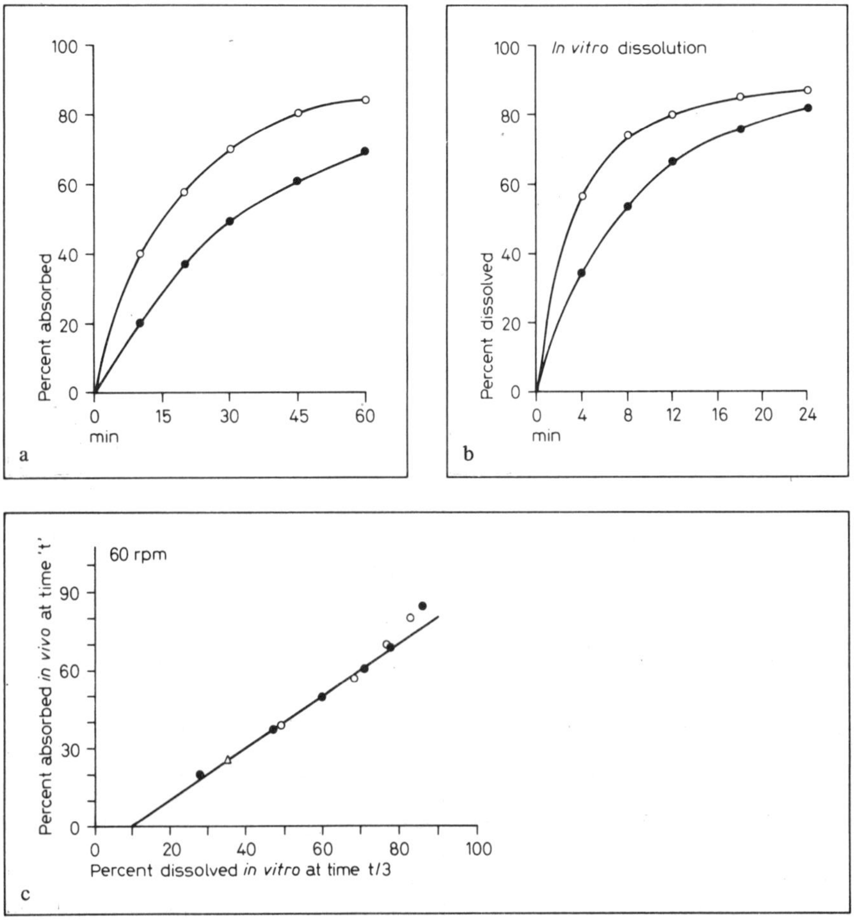

Fig. 27. Study 1: *in vitro/in vivo* correlation of buffered aspirin (○) and plain aspirin (●). Figures showing the percent absorbed with time following a 625-mg dose (a) and percent dissolved with time (b), in the beaker (0.1 N HCl, 250 ml, 60 rpm) and correlation between the amount absorbed at time (t) and amount dissolved *at a given time.* To obtain a slope of unity the *in vitro* amount dissolved was determined at time (t/3) (c) (103).

A second possibility is differences in *in vivo* absorption because of the larger dose given (large doses of aspirin may affect gastric emptying) or as suggested by *Levy* that these subjects were inexperienced and apprehension may have altered absorption. The latter possibility perhaps could be resolved if data were available on absorption from a solution.

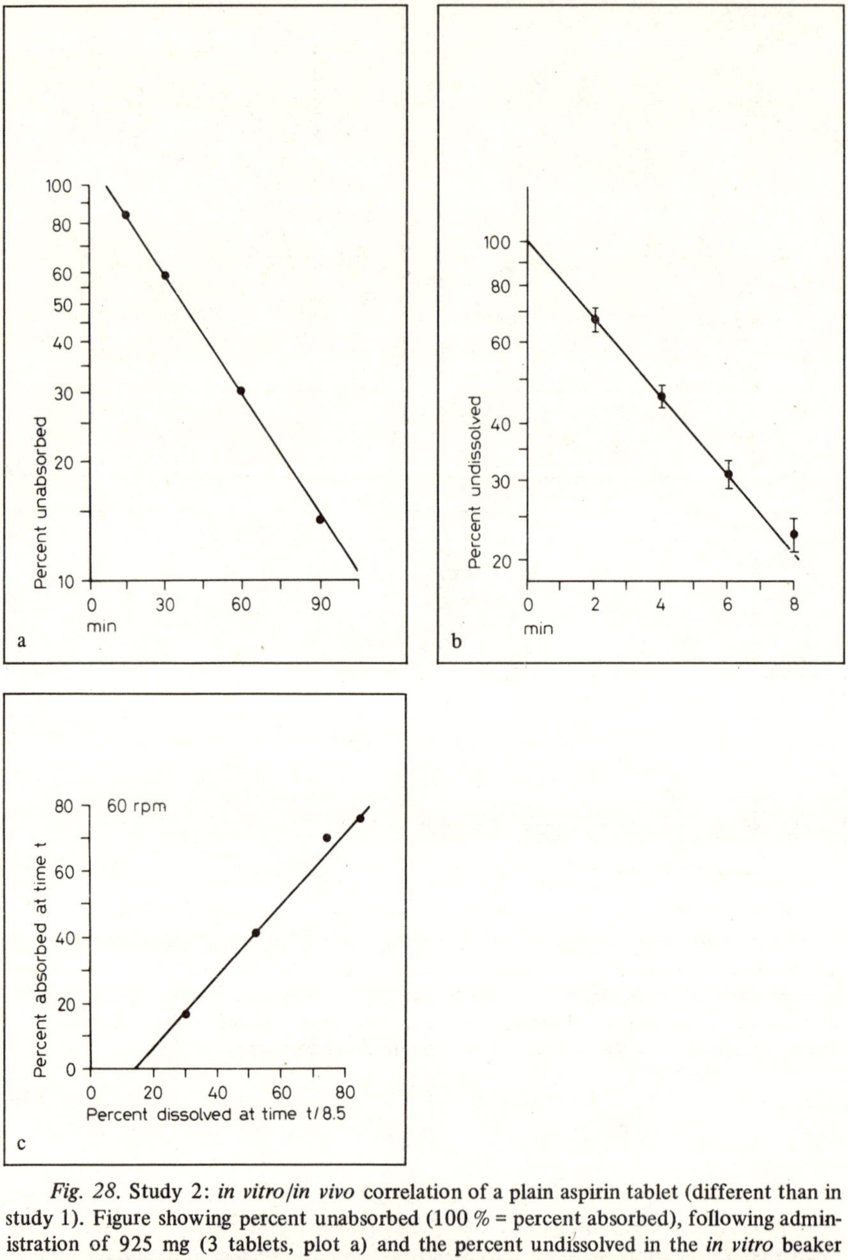

Fig. 28. Study 2: *in vitro/in vivo* correlation of a plain aspirin tablet (different than in study 1). Figure showing percent unabsorbed (100 % = percent absorbed), following administration of 925 mg (3 tablets, plot a) and the percent undissolved in the *in vitro* beaker method (0.1 N HCl, 350 ml, 60 rpm, in the plot b) and the correlation between the amount absorbed at time T and amount dissolved (plot c). To obtain a slope of unity the amounts dissolved were determined at time t/8.5 (104).

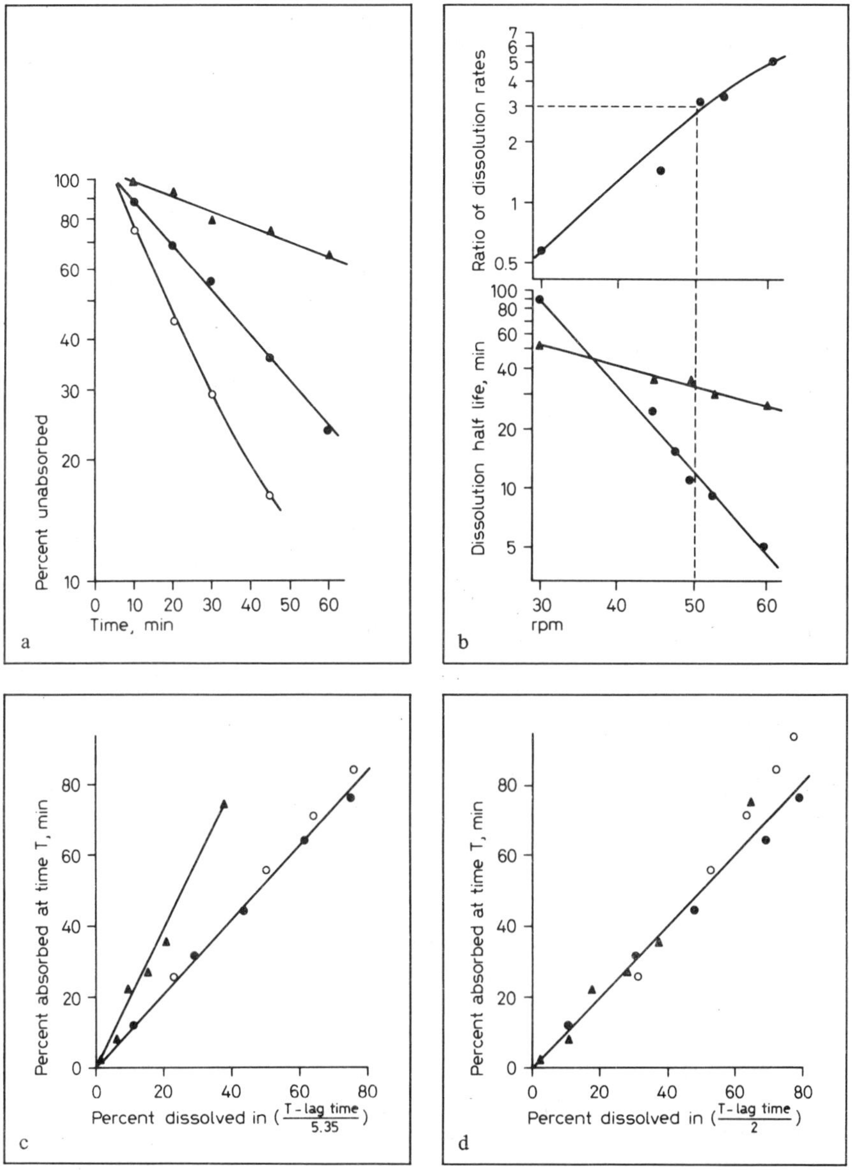

Fig. 29. Study 3: the *in vivo* absorption characteristics of a plain (●), buffered (○), and sustained release (▲) preparation (plot a), and the *in vitro* dissolution characteristics at different stirring rates (plot b), were correlated. Good correlation was obtained for the plain and buffered tablet at 60 rpm as in previous studies, but not the sustained release product (plot c). Good agreement for all three products was obtained only at 50 rpm (plot d) (105).

The third study involved the same brand of dosage forms as the first study with the addition of a sustained release product of microencapsulated particles. This study is quite comparable to the first. The same brands of plain and buffered aspirin were used, which *Levy* had shown previously that two lots of both these brands purchased a year apart, were essentially identical in their dissolution characteristics. Furthermore, the *in vivo* absorption rates of the solution, plain and buffered tablets were quite comparable to the previous study. As before, excellent correlation between the percent absorbed and percent dissolved with a stirring rate of 60 rpm for the buffered (B) and plain aspirin (A), which feil on the same regression line. However, the *in vivo/in vitro* slope for the microencapsulated product (C) was linear but had a different slope. As discussed before, this type of product is relatively independent of agitation intensities and thus should serve as marker to calibrate the *in vitro* stirring rate. The stirring rate which gave the same A/C ratio as the *in vivo* absorption rates was found to be 50 rpm. At this rate only did all products fall on the same regression line (fig. 29). Thus the diffusion rate-limited product (C) can serve as an 'internal marker' to adjust the stirring rate (105).

Although it would appear that 50 rpm seem to be the optimal stirring rate, a more recent study by *Levy* shows that life is not so simple. Two plain tablets were studied which differed only in the particle sizes of aspirin used in the formulation, one containing fine particles (< 80 mesh) and one containing coarse particles (> 20 mesh). The ratio of *in vivo* absorption rates of the product with fine particles to the product with large particles was 3:1. The *in vitro* dissolution rates at 50 rpm, however, was only 0.5. Only at a stirring rate of 55 does the ratio of *in vivo* rates of absorption equal the *in vitro* dissolution rates (fig. 30).

Weintraub and Gibaldi (102) have, from the previous data of *Levy et al.* (105), shown very good correlation between the amount dissolved in the rotating flask procedure and the amount absorbed for the plain, buffered and microencapsulated products. The advantage with this method is that crossover effects between these products were not observed when different agitation rates were used, presumably because of the better dispersion in this procedure. The best correlation was obtained at 0.9 rpm with the addition of a surfactant (fig. 31). It is interesting, however, that the addition of surfactant at 0.9 rpm does result in a crossover in dissolution rates of a capsule preparation with both the plain and buffered tablet. Unfortunately, data on *in vivo* absorption of the capsule are not available and the advisability of adding surfactant when capsule preparations are also being evaluated cannot be discerned.

The inescapable conclusion is that there appears to be no apparatus, agitation intensity, pH or additive which will result in perfect correlation for all types of dosage forms, even for aspirin, which is one of the drugs most likely to succeed.

30
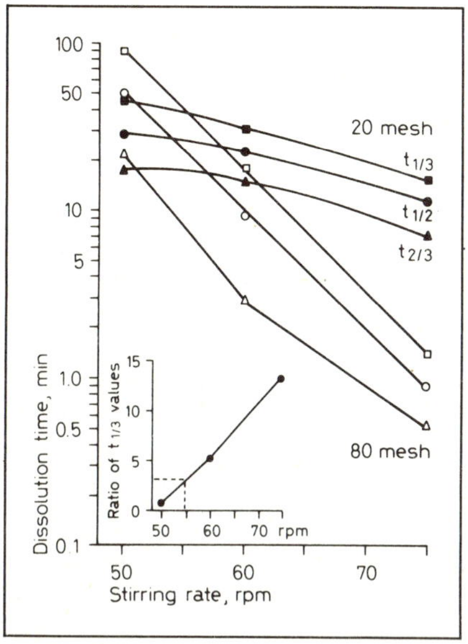

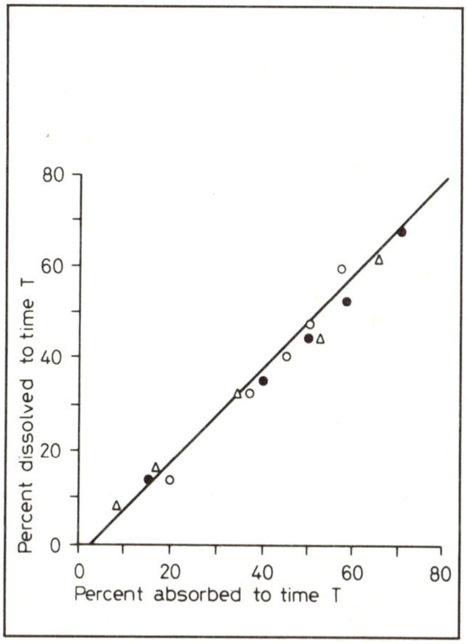

31

Fig. 30. Study 4: effect of agitation intensity on 'plain' aspirin products containing particles of 20 mesh (coarse, solid symbols) and 80 mesh (fine, open symbols). A 'crossover' in dissolution rates of the two products is seen at different agitation intensities. Only at rpm of 55 (interpolated, shown in the inset) does the ratio between the dissolution rates of the two products agree with the observed differences in absorption rates of the products (106). Squares = $t^1/_3$; circles = $t^1/_2$; triangles = $t^2/_3$.

Fig. 31. Relationship between percent aspirin dissolved and percent aspirin absorbed to the same time T. Dissolution data obtained in 0.1 N HCl with 0.01 % polyoxyethylene lauryl ether at 0.9 rpm in the rotating flask. Buffered tablets (○); plain tablets (●), and timed-release tablets (▲) (102).

Use of *in vitro* Dissolution Tests for Compendial Standards

There are now many drugs whose absorption characteristics have been shown to be related to and in some cases correlated with the dissolution characteristics of the dosage form. For drugs which have exhibited dissolution rate-dependent absorption it is necessary to develop *in vitro* dissolution tests which show the greatest sensitivity consistent with correlation to *in vivo* studies in man.

In vitro dissolution methodology will never exactly simulate the human intestine and never replace *in vivo* testing. It should neither be assumed or implied to be an absolute assessment of bioavailability. Its function as a compendial standard should be precisely that of its predecessor, the disintegration test, which is a quality control test that provides greater (but not absolute) assurance that the drug will be satisfactorily released from the dosage form *in vivo* and subsequently will be absorbed. If a product passes an *in vitro* dissolution test, it is not an absolute guarantee that the product will be well absorbed. If the product shows dissolution characteristics below certain limits by an appropriate method, then there is an increased probability that it will not be absorbed adequately and should be rejected unless acceptable bioavailability is shown by the primary standard.

Undoubtedly the greatest difficulty that we will face in establishing *in vitro* standards will be decisions on acceptable limits. For example, returning to the examples of drugs previously discussed, I am confident that we presently have sufficient information to develop standards which assure comparable absorption characteristics of aspirin products. However, I do not believe that anyone can presently tell us what differences in absorption rate will be clinically significant.

In the case of tetracycline I am confident that one could devise *in vitro* dissolution tests that would exclude virtually all products which would show clinically significant decreases in the amount of drug absorbed. I would not know where to set the limits to avoid excluding some products which would be acceptable.

Finally in the case of salicylamide, despite reports of apparent correlations between *in vitro* dissolution and total bioavailability, I do not believe that current information on desired *in vitro* dissolution characteristics is sufficient to allow any predictions on the rate and amount of *unmetabolized parent drug* which will reach the systemic circulation from various dosage forms.

Conclusions and Summary

The foregoing examples of the advantages and limitations of various types of methodology when applied to different uses in evaluating various drugs represent only a small sample of the available literature. Many other extensively studied drugs, such as griseofulvin, hydrochlorothiazide, phenylbutazone, warfarin, tolbutamide, and several others, would have served equally well to illustrate the basic points.

The examples given were intended to provide a basis for some conclusions and opinions summarized below:

1. There is a need to establish both primary and secondary types of standards which can be used by manufacturers, regulatory agencies, and practioners to evaluate the comparative performance of drugs which have exhibited a potential for clinical inequivalencies due to formulation variables.

2. The primary standard will usually be based on direct assessments of bioavailability (rate and extent) in man, by blood level and urinary excretion studies based on the best available analytical, pharmacokinetic and clinical

knowledge of the drug. This method will serve as the final criteria by which the second type of standard is developed. The secondary standard should be a relatively rapid, sensitive and reproducible method which does not require human experimentation but has demonstrated sensitivity to detect dosage forms which have significant potential to exhibit inadequate bioavailability by the primary standard. Results from the secondary standard are not to be assumed to be directly equated to bioavailability but rather as a quality control method which can screen out most undesirable products but not those which would be acceptable by the primary standard.

3. The rate of development and degree of success of methods to assess bioavailability of a specific drug will be directly proportional to the knowledge of the mechanisms involved in the interaction between the physiological variables of the absorption process and the physicochemical variables of the dosage form. The failure of most unsuccessful methods can frequently be attributed to lack of this knowledge.

4. *In vitro* and *in situ* preparations and studies, in intact and surgically manipulated small and larger animals, provide a variety of methods to study basic mechanisms of absorption of drugs from solid dosage forms. The use of larger animals, such as the dog or miniature pig, may serve as a useful screening method in the development of new dosage forms but in the opinion of this reviewer, an attempt to use them as a secondary standard is premature. There is presently not sufficient evidence of correlation between man and dog, pig or monkey, to compensate for the increased variability of animal testing and the considerable effort involved in collecting and analyzing biological fluids compared to physical methods. Development of simpler, more reproducible *in vitro* dissolution rate methods, which show reasonable correlation with the primary standard would appear to be the more expedient and fruitful initial approach to develop secondary standards.

5. The use of *in vitro* dissolution procedures as a secondary standard will depend on the sensitivity and degree of *in vivo* correlation with the primary standard. Several studies indicate that *in vitro* methods showing greatest sensitivity may be different from those showing the best *in vivo* correlation. The sensitivity and *in vivo* correlation of any *in vitro* method will be dependent on the release characteristics and other formulation variables of dosage form as well as the properties of drug studied. It will be more difficult to find a method which is applicable to all types of dosage forms than one suitable for one type or brand of dosage form. Consequently, there are two approaches which might be considered to establish secondary standards using *in vitro* physical methods.

(a) Since it may be possible for a manufacturer to establish an *in vitro* method showing excellent *in vivo* correlation for his product, even though the method may not be satisfactory to use as a general method for all other products, a suitable type of standard might be the *criteria* (e.g. precision reproducibility and sensitivity) required to establish that the correlation between the proposed secondary method and the critical *in vivo* parameter (e.g. rate, extent, peak blood level, etc.) is sufficient. For example, the manufacture could demonstrate that an *in vitro* method would distinguish between a series of products in which the critical formulation variables have been purposely varied to result in graded decreases in bioavailability determined by the primary standard. A 'standard curve' showing the degree of correlation between the secondary procedure and primary *in vivo* bioavailability could be constructed and evaluated by the criteria specified in the official standard. This is analogous to the accepted practice in which a manufacture may use an analytical procedure different from the official one, provided that it can be validated by standard curves with known concentrations showing at least comparable specificity and sensitivity. In these cases the burden of proof is with the manufacturer.

(b) The second approach would be to designate the specific type of apparatus and operation conditions to be used for all products without prior need by the manufacturer to establish *in vivo* correlation. There are several difficulties inherent in any attempt to develop such a general method and the requirements of such a method may be more involved.

6. It is the opinion of the author that attainment of a single 'universal dissolution method' is not a reasonable goal. It is more likely a myth which is intriguing to the imagination but has little basis in scientific fact. The closest thing to a perfect dissolution 'apparatus' would be the 'average gastrointestinal tracts' of a sufficiently large population to reflect normal variations. Even so, this 'apparatus' may not reflect significant clinical differences between two products in some patients with altered gastrointestinal function. A secondary *in vitro* standard generally useful to detect significant differences in many different brands may, therefore, require that a given dosage form be tested in more than one condition, for example, at different pH values, different agitation intensities or different types of agitation, in the presence and absence of surfactants or other additives, in 'sink' or non-'sink' conditions, or perhaps in different types of apparatus. In almost all cases it will be necessary to sample at more than one time-point to provide a better characterization of the entire dissolution curve than single-point determination (e.g. t_{50}).

7. Although development of a perfect dissolution procedure is highly unlikely, there is no doubt that improvement over present methods is quite possible and highly desirable. There is increasing evidence that the intrinsic hydrodynamic characteristics of the two methods presently official, have theoretical and practical shortcomings. The literature suggests that some desirable characteristics of new types of apparatus might include many of the following: (a) highly reproducible agitation rates that can be precisely controlled and quantitated over a wide range of very gentle to moderately intense agitation intensities; (b) the primary particles of the dosage form should be adequately dispersed at low

agitation intensities similar to dispersion *in vivo;* (c) abrasion of the dosage form or particles by the surfaces of the apparatus should be minimal; (d) the volume of the solvent should be capable of being varied over a sufficiently large range to provide 'sink' conditions for very insoluble drugs; (e) the solvent should be easily removed or exchanged to provide continuous or intermittent changes in pH, content of surfactants, enzymes, or other additives during the dissolution process; (f) the contents of the apparatus should be easily sampled, ideally by automated techniques without interrupting the dissolution process; (g) standardized parts should easily be attainable and relatively inexpensive, and (h) most important, the procedure should be very sensitive to small differences in dissolution characteristics in different types of dosage forms and show good correlation to the parameters of the primary *in vivo* method to assess bioavailability in man.

8. The difficulty in applying current information to develop better methodology to serve as secondary standards is that although there have been literally hundreds of studies reported, most have used different drugs, dosage forms, agitation intensities or different types of apparatus. Many studies provide no data in man to assess the predictive potential of the method used. There is, therefore, a mass of data which have no common means of comparison. When one considers the combinations and permutations of all possible drugs and conditions, it is quite possible that we may spend the next decade filling the literature with isolated studies and still not have an adequate dissolution standard for many drugs.

Attempts at interpretation, let alone correlation, of the voluminous published data on dissolution rates of different dosage form and of different apparatus using different conditions is frustrating, if not futile. Correlation of the results of future studies by different investigators will equally be frustrated unless some common denominator is provided.

What is presently needed is a series of reference dosage forms which can be used to calibrate different *in vivo* methods and serve as a basis of comparison for *in vitro* and *in vivo* studies of other products. Ideally, the reference series should have the following properties: (1) the reference dosage forms should cover a range of dissolution and absorption characteristics including a product which by current standards represents an acceptable formulation in terms of rate and extent of bioavailability; (2) the extent and rate of absorption of the products should be characterized in a large number of subjects (at least 20–30) using a protocol designed by a panel of experts in statistics and pharmacokinetics. Individual and group results should be available; (3) the dissolution characteristics in at least two standard methods should be available; (4) large quantities of the products should be available and easily duplicated, and (5) periodic quality control tests should be performed to assume that absorption and dissolution characteristics remain constant.

The standard reference dosage forms would serve several useful purposes: (1) to calibrate standard dissolution methods; (2) to evaluate and characterize new dissolution procedures; (3) to evaluate animal models for correlation; (4) the best product of a series could be used as the standard preparation in routine crossover studies to evaluate commercial products for regulatory or quality control purpose, and (5) the studies in normal subjects would provide the control data in evaluations of absorption of the drug and dosage forms in a variety of disease states.

The availability of a standard series which have been completely characterized in man would greatly reduce the expense and duplication involved if every investigator has to undergo extensive human bioavailability studies. Frequently such an extensive study in human subjects is beyond the capabilities of many investigators, which results in presentation of *in vitro* data only. Most important, a standard series would provide the means for direct comparison of studies from different laboratories using different *in vitro* methods, different animals, or disease conditions. The effort expended in developing such a series will be many times rewarded when our individual research efforts can be directly compared through a common denominator.

This is not a revolutionary suggestion. The USP has for several years recognized the need to supply reference standards of pure substances. It is a logical extension to apply the organizational and scientific expertise of this group perhaps in cooperation with other agencies such as the NF, FDA, FDD or manufacturers to developing reference standards for dosage forms. In my opinion this service is urgently needed to provide us with the standardized tools to develop a systematic approach to compare different *in vitro*, animal and human studies. I believe that such an approach will greatly accelerate our present task of finding the most effective and efficient means to provide uniform and optimal absorption characteristics of important therapeutic agents.

References

1 *Crane, R.K. and Wilson, T.H.:* J. appl. Physiol. *12:* 145 (1958).
2 *Shanker, L.S. and Tocco, D.J.:* J. Pharmacol. exp. Ther. *123:* 8 (1960).
3 *Aguiar, A.J. and Fifelski, R.J.:* J. pharm. Sci. *55:* 1387 (1966).
4 *Taraszka, M.J.:* J. pharm. Sci. *60:* 946 (1971).
5 *Reuning, R. and Levy, G.:* J. pharm. Sci. *57:* 1335 (1968).
6 *Aguiar, A.:* Drug Inform. Bull. *3:* 17 (1969).
7 *Reuning, R. and Levy, G.:* J. pharm. Sci. *57:* 1342 (1968).
8 *Feldman, S. and Gibaldi, M.:* J. pharm. Sci. *58:* 425 (1969).
9 *Saski, W.:* J. pharm. Sci. *57:* 836 (1968).
10 *Benet, L.Z.; Orr, J.M.; Turner, R.H., and Webb, H.S.:* J. pharm. Sci. *60:* 234 (1971).
11 *Mayersohn, M. and Gibaldi, M.:* J. pharm. Sci. *60;* 225 (1971).

12 *Strahl, N.:* Kinetics and mechanisms of aryl acid transport across the rat intestine; Ph.D. thesis, Buffalo (1971).
13 *Levy, G. and Angelino, N.J.:* J. pharm. Sci. *57:* 1449 (1968).
14 *Strahl, N. and Barr, W.H.:* J. pharm. Sci. *60:* 278 (1971).
15 *Barr, W.H. and Riegelman, S.:* J. pharm. Sci. *59:* 154 (1970).
16 *Barr, W.H. and Riegelman, S.:* J. pharm. Sci. *59:* 164 (1970).
17 *Chung, M. and Barr, W.H.:* (unpublished data).
18 *Feldman, S.; Salvino, M., and Gibaldi, M.:* J. pharm. Sci. *59:* 705 (1970).
19 *Shanker, L.:* J. med. Chem. *2:* 343 (1970).
20 *Hogben, C.A.M.; Tocco, D.J.; Brodie, B.B., and Schanker, L.:* J. Pharmacol. exp. Therap. *125:* 275 (1959).
21 *Kakemi, K.; Arita, T.; Hori, R., and Konishi, K.:* Chem. pharm. Bull. *15:* 1534 (1967).
22 *Shedle, H.P.:* J. clin. Endocrin. Metab. *25:* 1309 (1965).
23 *Doluisio, J.T.; Bellups, N.F.; Dittert, L.W.; Sugita, E.J., and Swintowsky, J.V.:* J. pharm. Sci. *58:* 1196 (1969).
24 *Ho, N.F.; Higuchi, W.I., and Doluisio, J.T.:* to be published.
25 *Oshenfarhrt, O. and Winne, D.:* Life Sci. *7:* 493 (1968).
26 *Pindall, M.H.; Cull, K.M.; Doran, K.M., and Dickenson, H.L.:* J. Pharmacol. exp. Ther. *125:* 287 (1959).
27 *Sturtevant, F.M.; Pauls, J.F., and Abrams:* Toxicol. appl. Pharmacol. *3:* 80 (1961).
28 *Morozowich, W.; Chulski, T.; Hamlin, W.E.; Jones, P.M.; Northam, J.I.; Purmalio, A., and Wagner, J.G.:* J. pharm. Sci. *51:* 993 (1962).
29 *Dittert, L.; Adams, H.; Alexander, F.; Chong, C.; Ellison, T., and Swintowski, J.V.:* J. pharm. Sci. *57:* 1146 (1968).
30 *Mullins, J. and Macek, T.J.:* Amer. pharm. Ass. Sci. Ed. *49:* 245 (1960).
31 *Lee, C.; Froman, R.O.; Anderson, R.C., and Chen, K.K.:* Antibiot. Chemother. N.Y. *8:* 354 (1958).
32 *Harris, P.A. and Riegelman, S.:* J. pharm. Sci. *58:* 71 (1969).
33 *Synchowicz, S.; Zeman, W.V.; Williams, R.A., and Tabachnick, I.I.A.:* Arch. int. Pharmacodyn. *158:* 360 (1965).
34 *Lackman, L.; Barrett, W.; Rinehard, R.K., and Sheppard, H.:* Curr. Therap. Res. *6:* 491 (1964).
35 *Sample, R.G.; Rossi, G.V., and Packman, E.W.:* J. pharm. Sci. *57:* 795 (1968).
36 *Poole, J.W.:* Drug Inform. Bull. *3:* 8 (1969).
37 *Cressman, W.A.; Janicki, C.A.; Johnson, P.C.; Doluisio, J.T., and Braun, G.A.:* J. pharm. Sci. *58:* 1516 (1969).
38 J. pharm. Sci. *56* (1967).
39 *Withey, R.:* Symposium on 'perspectives in bioavailability of drugs, therapeutic and toxicological significance', Canad. Ass. Res. in Toxicology, Montreal 1971, and personal communication.
40 *Weiner, M.:* Paper presented to 1971 National Industrial Pharmaceutical Research Conference, 'Drug absorption through the gastrointestinal barrier', Land O'Lakes, Wisc.
41 *Aguiar, A.J.; Krc, J., jr.; Kinkel, A.W., and Samyn, J.C.:* J. pharm. Sci. *56:* 847 (1967).
42 *Bauer, G.; Rieckman, P., and Schaumann:* Arzneimittelforsch. *12:* 487 (1962).
43 *Kraml, M.; Dubuc, J., and Gaudry, R.:* Antibiot. Chemother. N.Y. *12:* 239 (1962).
44 *Marvel et al.:* J. invest. Derm. *37:* 1967 (1963).
45 *Wagner, J.G.:* Drug intelligence *3:* 198, 224, 278, 324, 357 (1969).
46 *Swarbrick, J.* (ed.): Current concepts in the pharmaceutical sciences (Lea & Febiger, Philadelphia 1970).
47 *Wood, J.:* Pharm. Acta Helv. *42:* 129 (1967).

48 *Higuchi, T.:* J. pharm. Sci. *56:* 315 (1967).
49 *Hersey, J.A.:* Mfg Chem. *40:* 32 (1969).
50 *Fincher, J.:* J. pharm. Sci. *57:* 1825 (1968).
51 *Wurster, D.E., and Taylor, P.W.:* J. pharm. Sci. *54:* 169 (1965).
52 *Niebergall, P.J.; Milosovich, G., and Goyan, J.E.:* J. pharm. Sci. *52:* 236 (1963).
53 *Higuchi, W.I.; Mir, N.A., and Desai, S.J.:* J. pharm. Sci. *54:* 1405 (1965).
54 *Nelson, E.; Knolchel, E.L.; Hamlin, W.E., and Wagner, J.G.:* J. pharm. Sci. *51:* 509 (1962).
55 *Nelson, E.:* Chem. pharm. Bull. *10:* 1099 (1962).
56 *Levy, G.; Antkowiak, J.M.; Prochnal, J.A., and White, D.C.:* *52:* 1047 (1963).
57 *Wood, J.:* J. pharm. Sci. *54:* 1207 (1965).
58 *Paikoff, M. and Drumm, G.:* J. pharm. Sci. *54:* 1693 (1965).
59 *Schroeter, L.C.; Tingstad, J.E.; Koechel, E.L., and Wagner, J.G.:* J. pharm. Sci. *51:* 865 (1962).
60 *Levy, G. and Hayes:* New Engl. J. Med. *262:* 1053 (1960).
61 *Morrison, A.B. and Campbell:* J. pharm. Sci. *54:* 1 (1965).
62 *Yen, J.K.C.:* Canad. pharm. J. *97:* 493 (1964).
63 *Kildig:* Proc. 5th Nat. Meet. APhA Acad. Pharm. Sci., Washington, D.C., 1970, p. 227.
64 *Campagna, J.; Cureton, G.; Mirigian, R., and Nelson, E.:* J. pharm. Sci. *52:* 605 (1963).
65 *Levy, G.:* Lancet (1962).
66 *Levy, G.:* Canad. med. Ass. J. *90:* 978 (1964).
67 *Keller, W.:* Pharmazie *15:* 56 (1960).
68 *Markus, A.:* Proc. 5th Nat. Meet. APhA Acad. Pharm. Sci., Washington, D.C., 1970, p. 291.
69 *Pernarowski:* ibid, p. 310.
70 United States Pharmacopeia XVIII, standards for hydrochlorthiazide, meprobamate, nitrofurantoin, prednisone, prednisolone, sulfisoxazole and tolbutamide.
71 National Formulary XVIII, standards for acetohexamide, methandrostenolone, sulfamethoxazole and methylprednisolone.
72 *Barr, W.H.; Letcher, K., and Adir, J.:* Abstracts of APhA Acad. Pharm. Sci. Ann. Meet., Washington, D.C., 1970.
73 *Barr, W.H.; Adir, J., and Garrettson, L.:* Clin. Pharmacol. Ther. *12:* 779 (1971).
74 *Nelson, E.:* J. amer. pharm. Ass. (Sci. Ed.) *48:* 96 (1959).
75 *Macdonald, H.; Pisano, F.; Burger, J.; Dornbush, A., and Pelcak, E.:* Drug Inform. Bull. *3:* 76 (1969).
76 *Barr, W.H.:* Drug Inform. Bull. *3:* 27 (1969).
77 *Barr, W.H.; Gerbracht, L.; Letcher, K.; Plaut, M., and Strahl, N.R.:* Clin. Pharmacol. Ther. (in press).
78 *O'Reilly, R.A.; Nelson, E., and Levy, G.:* J. pharm. Sci. *55:* 435 (1966).
79 *Riegelman, S.:* Drug Inform. Bull. *3:* 59 (1969).
80 *Adir, J. and Barr, W.H.:* to be published.
81 *Krauer, B. and Dettli, L.:* Chemotherapia *14:* 1 (1969).
82 *Dettli and Spring, P.:* Helv. med. Acta *33:* 291 (1966).
83 *Levy, G.:* J. pharm. Sci. *50:* 181 (1969).
84 *Bernard, B.; Yin, E.J., and Simon, H.J.:* J. clin. Pharmacol. *11:* 332 (1971).
85 *Barr, W.H. and Riegelman, S.:* to be published.
86 *Levy, G. and Matsuzawa, J.J.:* J. Pharmacol. exp. Ther. *156:* 285 (1967).
87 *Bates, T.R.; Lambert, D.A., and Johns, W.H.:* J. pharm. Sci. *58:* 1468 (1969).
88 *Barr, W.H.; Guzzo, G.; Aceto, T., jr., and Garrettson, L.:* Paper presented to the APhA Acad. Pharm. Sci., Washington, D.C., 1970.

89 *Nelson, E.:* J. amer. pharm. Ass. (Sci. Ed.) *47:* 297 (1958).
90 *Levy, G.:* J. pharm. Sci. *52:* 1039 (1963).
91 *Ballard, B.E. and Biles, J.A.:* Steroids *4:* 273 (1964).
92 *Levy, G. and Hayes, B.A.:* New Engl. J. Med. *21:* 1053 (1960).
93 *Parrott, E.L.; Wurster, D.E., and Higuchi, T.:* J. amer. pharm. Ass. (Sci. Ed.) *44:* 269 (1955).
94 *Wood, J.; Syarto, J.E.; Syarto, L.C., and Herman, H.:* J. pharm. Sci. *54:* 1068 (1965).
95 *Pernarowski, M.; Woo, W., and Searl, R.O.:* J. pharm. Sci. *57:* 1419 (1968).
96 *Cook, D.; Chang, H.S., and Mainville, C.A.:* Canad. J. pharm. Sci. *2:* 91 (1966).
97 *Gibaldi, M. and Weintraub, H.:* J. pharm. Sci. *59:* 725 (1970).
98 *Braun, D.G. and Walker, G.C.:* J. pharm. Sci. *58:* 611 (1969).
99 *Wagner, J.G.:* Drug Intellig. and Clin. Pharm. *4:* 232 (1970).
100 *Levy, G.:* J. pharm. Sci. *52:* 1039 (1963).
101 *Levy, G.:* J. Mondial Pharm. (July–Sept.) 1967.
102 *Weintraub, H. and Gibaldi, M.:* J. pharm. Sci. *59:* 1792 (1970).
103 *Levy, G.:* Arch. Int. Pharmacodyn. *152:* 59 (1964).
104 *Levy and Hollister, L.E.:* J. pharm. Sci. *53:* 1446 (1964).
105 *Levy, G.; Leonards, J.R., and Prochnal, J.A.:* J. pharm. Sci. *54:* 1719 (1965).
106 *Levy, G.; Leonards, J.R., and Prochnal, J.A.:* J. pharm. Sci. *56:* 1365 (1967).

Author's address: Prof. *William H. Barr,* Department of Pharmaceutics, State University of New York, *Buffalo, NY 14214* (USA)

Pharmacology *8:* 102–117 (1972)

An Overview of the Analysis and Interpretation of Bioavailability Studies in Man

J.G. Wagner

University Hospital, The University of Michigan, Ann Arbor, Mich.

Introduction

This is a conference on bioavailability of drugs. A major reason for the need for bioavailability studies has roots in the generic equivalence and inequivalence problem. I would like to make some brief introductory remarks about this problem before pursuing my major assignment.

There are a few people in this audience and elsewhere who continue to say there really is not a generic equivalence and inequivalence problem. In a chapter in my new textbook (1) I discuss generic equivalence and inequivalence of oral products and clearly point out that, where carefully controlled clinical studies have been carried out, results have predominently shown *inequivalence.* Hence, this small sample – all the work that has been done – indicates that we do have a problem. I fail to understand how anyone can conclude that since all the other drugs, sold by more than one manufacturer, have not been studied, then they can be assumed to be equivalent. This seems to be the very opposite of what would be expected from statistical sampling techniques.

Perhaps there are some people who still question the importance and significance of bioavailability testing.

Table I summarizes results of *Manninen et al.* (2). 19 patients who were stabilized to digoxin, 0.25 mg, tablet 'A', were studied by measuring plasma levels of digoxin for a few days, then they were switched to brand 'B' tablets at the same label doses. The average plasma digoxin level rose by 48 % from 1.85 ng/ml to 2.74 ng/ml, and 3 patients showed signs of digitalis intoxication. After a period of 5 days on tablet 'B', the patients were switched back to tablet 'A' and, within 4 more days, the average plasma digoxin concentration decreased 40 % and came essentially to the same average as they had originally shown when given tablet 'A'. The authors concluded: 'If the patient is well established on a given preparation, unnecessary changes may increase the hazards of digoxin therapy and should be avoided. The costs of digoxin therapy are low for an individual patient, but for large-scale use the best absorbed preparation may be economically worth considering.' This was a fixed-dose study; it is obvious the patients taking tablet 'B' could get along very well by taking fewer digoxin tablets, or lower potency tablets, due to the improved absorption. Bioavailability of digoxin, particularly during digitalization, could mean life or death for a patient; hence, the problem is important. Some might say: 'But these tablets were made in Europe.' We have the same problem here in the US. The December 7, 1971 issue of the New England Journal of Medicine will verify my statement.

Recently there has been some talk of a cost/availability ratio among some poorly informed people. Data collected so far show that if a product is fully bioavailable, the bioavailability in different subjects and in the same subject at different times is within a very narrow range, say 95–100 %. However, if a poorly available product has an *average* bioavailability of say 50 %, the range in individual patients, and in the same patient at different times, covers a tremendous range, sometimes from 0 to 100 %! If a patient is chronically taking a cardiotonic glycoside, such as digoxin or digitoxin, he or she *needs* the entire dose of medicine every day, and not a variable amount or none at all, depending upon the particular tablet he ingests each day. Hence, those who are naive and discuss a cost/availability ratio should be well aware of this pitfall.

Finally, *Morris* (3), an attorney at law in Cleveland, Ohio, recently published an article entitled: 'R_X: brand or generic? Your decision may be important in a malpractice defense.' If I read this article correctly, it means that a practicing physician may be liable to his patient for a generic prescription he wrote, *even though* he was unaware of exactly which brand a pharmacist dispensed. The implications of this article are important for the physician and should be considered by the APhA in future discussions in the generic and antisubstitution law areas.

Table I. Average equilibrium state in 19 patients treated with digoxin

Digoxin treatment, 0.25 mg	Period	Digoxin plasma concentration, ng/ml	
Tablet 'A'	initial	1.85	
			Difference 0.89 or *48 %*
Tablet 'B'	middle	2.74	
			Difference 0.78 or *40 %*
Tablet 'A'	final	1.96	

'If the patient is well established on a given preparation, unnecessary changes may increase the hazards of digoxin in therapy and should be avoided. The costs of digoxin therapy are low for an individual patient, but for large-scale use the best absorbed preparations may be economically worth considering' (2).

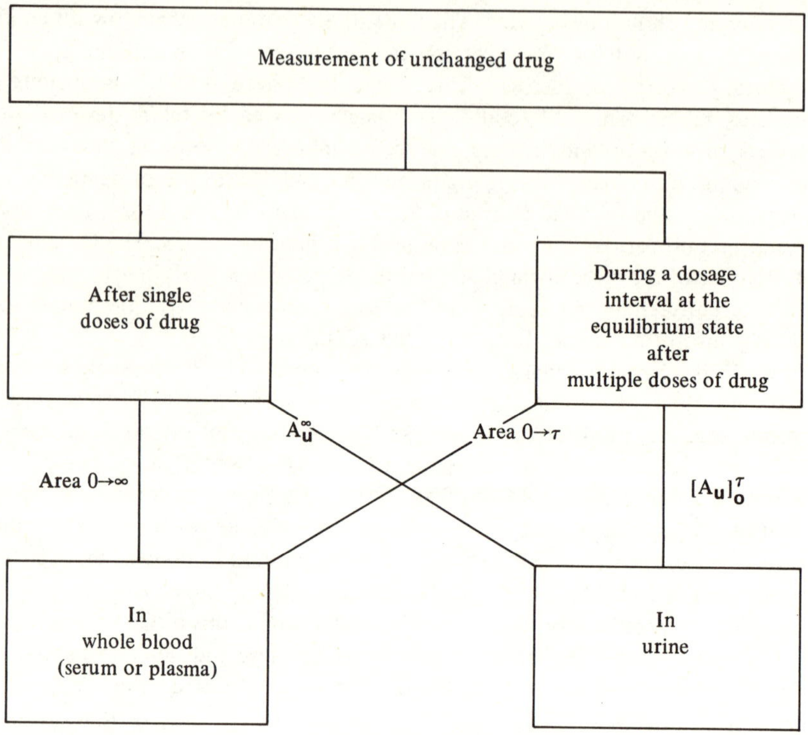

Fig. 1. Methods based on clinical studies in man where 'blood levels' and/or urinary excretion are measured.

Overview

Now, I will return to my assigned subject. I have summarized the different types of bioavailability studies, and the various methods of analysis and interpretation of data, in several tables and figures. The 'Glossary of Symbols' on pages 99–101 defines the different symbols shown in the tables and figures.

Figures 1, 2 and 3 summarize methods of estimation of bioavailability based on clinical studies in man where blood levels and/or urinary excretion are measured. Figure 1 considers measurement of unchanged drug. Figure 2 considers measurement of a metabolite of the drug. Figure 3 considers measurement of total drug (i.e. unchanged drug plus total metabolites). It should be noted that this does *not* include a case such as chlorpromazine where total so-called 'phenothiazine nucleus' accounts for only 15–50 % of the administered dose. Such an assay for determination of bioavailability is a problem from my point of view.

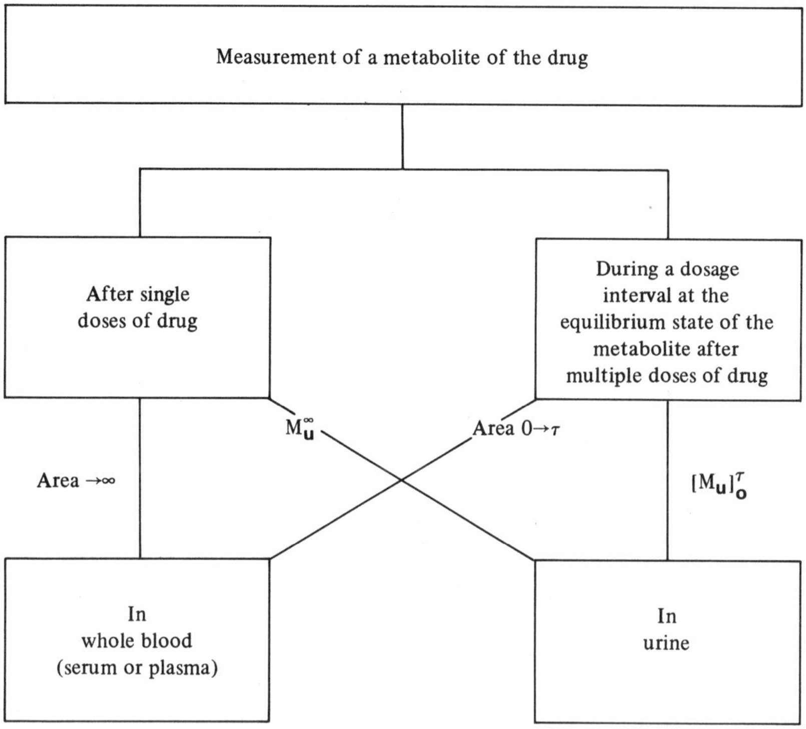

Fig. 2. Methods based on clinical studies in man where 'blood levels' and/or urinary excretion are measured.

Table II. Methods based on clinical trials

1. Some quantitative end-point, which measures efficacy of the drug or quantitates drug effect, should be used, e.g. blood sugar lowering by an anti-diabetic agent, blood pressure lowering produced by a hypotensive agent, or weight loss produced by an anorexagenic agent.
2. Prior information must include a satisfactory dose-response curve with a high r^2 value obtained with a known readily available or standard formulation of the drug.
3. Sufficient subjects or patients must be used to be able to show that a specified difference in extreme means (say 20 %) is significant at the $p = 0.05$ level with sufficient power ($1-\beta \simeq 0.6$ or 0.7).

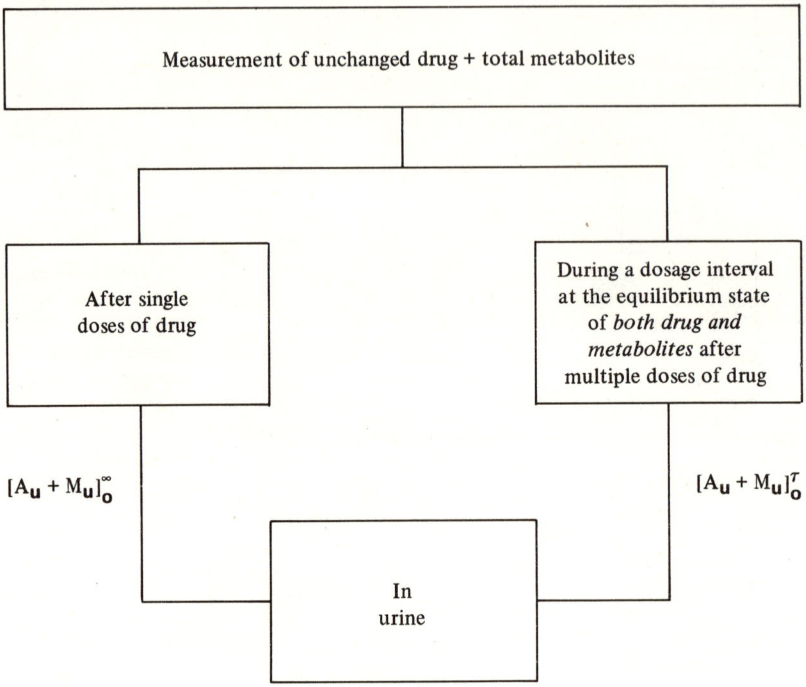

Fig. 3. Methods based on clinical studies in man where 'blood levels' and/or urinary excretion are measured.

Table III.

If clearance, dose, fraction of dose absorbed, and dosage interval $\tau = (t_2 - t_1)$ are constant for a multiple dose regimen, then:

$$\int_{t_1}^{t_2} C_\infty(t)dt = \int_0^\infty C(t)dt \qquad (1)$$

and

either area will be a linear function of dose (2)

providing·

(1) the system may be described by a system of linear differential equations,

or

(2) the system may be described by a system of nonlinear differential equations for a mammilary model in which the exit rate constant is a first order rate constant.

Neither 1 or 2 will hold if there is a nonlinear system involving the exit of the drug (e.g. *Michaelis-Menten* kinetics) and the concentrations are above the first-order region.

Table IV. Single dose case measurement of unchanged drug excreted in the urine in 'infinite time' (about 7–10 half-lives of the drug)

If $(\overline{A_u^\infty})_A - (\overline{A^\infty})_B$ is significant at $p \leq 0.05$, then

$$\frac{(\overline{A_u^\infty})_B}{(\overline{A_u^\infty})_A} = \frac{\bar{f}_B \bar{F}_B \bar{D}_B}{\bar{f}_A \bar{F}_A \bar{D}_A} = \frac{\bar{F}_B}{\bar{F}_A}$$

providing that:

(1) $\bar{D}_B = \bar{D}_A$ (if not, a correction for dose is made)

(2) $\bar{f}_B = \bar{f}_A$

when drug is administered intravenously then:

$$f = \frac{A_u^\infty}{D}$$

After oral or intravenous administration:

$$f = \frac{A_u^\infty}{A_u^\infty + M_{ui}^\infty + \text{---------} + M_{un}^\infty}$$

and

$$f = \frac{k_d}{k_d + k_{fi} + \text{---------} + k_{fn}} = \frac{k_d}{k_{el}}$$

Multiple Dose Case

$[\overline{A_u}]_0^\tau$ replaces $\overline{A_u^\infty}$ and need only collect urine in one dosage interval at equilibrium state.

Table II discusses methods based on clinical trials. Points 2 and 3 in table II are worthy of note. Methods based on clinical trials are really of no value, and give meaningless answers, unless these points are met.

Table III discusses the pharmacokinetic principle which allows us to compare blood levels following single doses and those obtained after multiple doses at the equilibrium state. The area relationship is valid in some nonlinear cases as well as all linear cases.

Table IV discusses the pharmacokinetic principle behind estimation of drug availability by measuring unchanged drug excreted in urine following single and multiple doses of drug in crossover studies. Note that urine must be collected for at least seven elimination half-lives of drug in order for the method to be valid. 24- or 48-hour urine collections are just not good enough unless the elimination half-life of the drug is small.

Table V. Single dose case measurement of amount of a metabolite excreted in the urine in 'infinite time' (about 7–10 half-lives of the metabolite)

If $(\overline{M_{ui}^{\infty}})_A - (\overline{M_{ui}^{\infty}})_B$ is significant at $p = \leq 0.05$, then

$$\frac{(\overline{M_{ui}^{\infty}})_B}{(\overline{M_{ui}^{\infty}})_A} = \frac{(\overline{f_{mi}}) \cdot F_B \cdot D_B}{(\overline{f_{mi}}) \cdot F_A \cdot D_A} = \frac{\overline{F_B}}{\overline{F_A}}$$

providing that:

(1) $\bar{D}_B = \bar{D}_A$ (if not, a correction for dose is made).

(2) $(\overline{f_{mi}})_B = (\overline{f_{mi}})_A$

when the drug is given intravenously then:

$$f = \frac{M_{ui}^{\infty}}{D}$$

After oral or intravenous administration:

$$f_{mi} = \frac{M_{ui}^{\infty}}{A_u^{\infty} + M_{ui}^{\infty} + -------- + M_{un}^{\infty}}$$

and

$$f_{mi} = \frac{k_f}{k_d + k_f + -------- + k_{fn}} = \frac{k_{fi}}{k_{el}}$$

Multiple Dose Case

$(\overline{M_{ui}})_0^{\tau}$ replaces $\overline{M_{ui}^{\infty}}$ and need only collect urine in one dosage interval at equilibrium state.

Table V covers measurement of a metabolite of the drug in urine.

Table VI discusses the method of *Wagner* (4) as applied to blood-level data. The ratios shown on the left-hand side of the third or sixth equation are calculated from the data for each subject on each treatment in a crossover study, then the values of the ratios are analyzed by analysis of variance for crossover design.

Table VII covers methods of estimation of bioavailability based on area measurements. Methods A, B and D are applied to crossover studies. Method C applies to noncrossover studies, but it should be noted that one probably never gets the correct answer in noncrossover studies, since the answers are biased by the means and standard deviations of the distributions of the volumes of distribution in the two panels of subjects.

Table VI. Method of *Wagner*

One-compartment open model interpretation

$$F \cdot D = V \cdot K \cdot A$$

$$F \cdot \frac{D}{W} = \frac{V}{W} \cdot K \cdot A$$

$$\frac{K \cdot A}{(D/W)} = \frac{0.693A}{(T\frac{1}{2})\,(D/W)} = \frac{F}{(V/W)}$$

Two-compartment open model interpretation

$$F \cdot D = V_p \cdot k_{el} \cdot A = V_{d_{area}} \cdot \beta \cdot A$$

$$F \cdot \frac{D}{W} = \frac{V_{d_{area}}}{W} \cdot \beta \cdot A$$

$$\frac{\beta \cdot A}{(D/W)} = \frac{0.693A}{(T\frac{1}{2})\,(D/W)} = \frac{F}{(V_{d_{area}}/W)}$$

The constant clearance method using uncorrected areas assumes $(V_p \cdot k_{el}/W)$ is constant intrasubject whereas this method assumes $(V_p \cdot k_{el}/W \cdot \beta)$ is constant intrasubject.

Table VII. Extent of bioavailability based on area measurements

A. If clearance and dose constant and crossover study, then percent availability of 'B' relative to 'A' = $(A_B/A_A) \times 100$.
B. If clearance constant and crossover study, but doses different, then: percent availability of 'B' relative to 'A' = $(A_B/A_A) \times (D_A/D_B) \times 100$.
C. If clearance constant, doses are different and noncrossover study with two different groups of subjects given the two treatments, then: percent availability of 'B' relative to 'A' = $(A_B/A_A) \times (D_A/D_B) \times (W_B/W_A) \times 100$.

but the answer is biased since it depends upon the means and standard deviations of the distributions of volumes of distributions in the two panels of subjects.
D. If rate constant (β) estimated from terminal blood levels or elimination half-life ($\ln 2/\beta$) varies intrasubject, then percent availability of 'B' relative to 'A'

$$(\beta_B \cdot A_B/\beta_A \cdot A_A) \cdot (D_A/D_B) = ([T\tfrac{1}{2}]_A \cdot A_B \cdot D_A/[T\tfrac{1}{2}]_B \cdot A_A \cdot D_B)$$

In the above: $A = \int_0^{\infty} C(t)dt$ or $A = \int_{t_1}^{t_2} C_{\infty}(t)dt$

Table VIII. Method of *Loo and Riegelman*

This method assumes that the two-compartment open model applies.
1. Drug administered intravenously and concentration data fitted to:

$$C_p = \frac{D}{V_p(\alpha-\beta)}\left[(k_{21}-\beta)e^{-\beta t}-(k_{21}-\alpha)e^{-\alpha t}\right]$$

where $\alpha + \beta = k_{12} + k_{21} + k_{el}$ and $\alpha \cdot \beta = k_{21}\, k_{el}$

2. Drug administered orally and following equation applied:

$$\text{(a)}\quad (A/V_p)_{tn} = (C_p)_{tn} + k_{el}\int_0^{tn} C_1\,(t)dt + (C_t)_{tn}$$

where

$$(C_t)_{tn} = (C_p)_{tn-1} \cdot e^{-k_{21}\Delta t} + \frac{k_{12}}{k_{21}}(C_p)_{tn-1}\left[1-e^{-k_{21}\Delta t}\right] + \frac{k_{12}\Delta C_p \Delta t}{2}$$

where k_{12} and k_{21} are the same as in i.v. study, and k_{el} is the same or a new value calculated from new β value.

(b) The asymptote of a plot of $(A/V_p)_{tn}$ *versus* t is $k_{el}\int_0^\infty C_p\,(t)dt$,

hence

$$\%\ \text{absorbed} = \frac{(A/V_p)_{tn}}{k_{el}\int_0^\infty C_p\,(t)dt} \times 100$$

Hence this method provides:
I. An estimate of absolute efficiency of absorption.
II. A plot of cumulative percent absorbed versus time which may be resolved to indicate the kinetics of absorption.

Table VIII covers the method of *Loo and Riegelman* (5). There are several variations of this method – a recent one allowing one to make a correction if the value of β changes in a subject from intravenous to oral administration. The method provides: (1) an estimate of absolute efficiency of absorption, and (2) a plot of cumulative percent absorbed versus time which may be resolvable to indicate the kinetics of absorption.

Table IX summarizes some of the pitfalls of the pharmacokinetic methods.

Table X takes a simple pharmacokinetic model and shows why the time of the peak blood level and the value of the peak blood level *may be* indicators of drug availability. A pitfall is discussed at the bottom of table X.

Table IX. Pitfalls in methods based on measurement of drug and metabolites in blood and urine

---

1. You must estimate the *total* area under the curve and you must collect urine long enough to measure *all* the compound excreted in urine.
2. In application of both the *Wagner* method and the *Loo and Riegelman* method, concentrations must be measured long enough that $\hat{\beta}$ is not appreciably affected by continued absorption of the drug.
3. With shorter half-life drugs, the 'flip-flop' model is possible where terminal concentration data yield the absorption rate constant(s).
4. If there is a 'first pass' effect then $A_{oral} < A_{i.v.}$
5. Estimation of the area $T \rightarrow \infty$ (where T is last sampling time) after single doses is model dependent. The area $0 \rightarrow \tau$ after multiple doses is *not* similarly dependent.
6. When k_{21} is approximately equal to either α or one (or the only) input rate constants, then one exponential term describing oral data will be essentially zero and erroneous answers are obtained.

Table X. Why 'time of peak blood level' and 'peak blood level' may be indicators of extent of bioavailability

---

$$\left\langle C_0 = \frac{FD}{V} \right\rangle \xrightarrow{\quad k \quad} \boxed{V} \xrightarrow{\quad K \quad}$$

$$C = C_0\left(\frac{\gamma}{\gamma-1}\right)\left[2^{-n} - 2^{-\gamma n}\right] \text{ where } n = t/t_{1/2} \text{ and } \gamma = k/K$$

$$\int_0^N C \cdot dn = \frac{C_0}{\ln 2}\left[1 - \frac{1}{\gamma-1}\left\langle \gamma 2^{-n} - 2^{-\gamma n} \right\rangle\right]$$

$$\int_0^\infty C dn = \frac{C_0}{\ln 2}$$

$$n_{max} = \frac{t\ max}{t_{\frac{1}{2}}} = \frac{\ln \gamma}{\ln 2\ (\gamma - 1)}$$

$$C\ max = C_0 \gamma^{(1/1-\gamma)}$$

If $N \geq 2$ and $\gamma \geq 5$:

(a) Will find for group of subjects given different dosage forms of a drug or the same dosage form that any pair of $\int_0^N Cdn$, $\int_0^\infty Cdn$, n_{max}, and C max are highly correlated.

(b) Similarly, $\int_0^{t \geq 2t_{\frac{1}{2}}} Cdt$, $\int_0^\infty Cdt$, t max and C max will be highly correlated.

Pitfall

When γ varies widely from dosage form to dosage form, one can have the areas essentially equal, but the peaks and peak times vary widely.

Table XI. Areas 0→n[1], where n is the number of half-lives of elimination for one-compartment open model with first-order absorption[2]

n	$\gamma = \frac{\text{rate constant for absorption}}{\text{rate constant for alimination}}$				
	100.0	10.0	5.0	2.0	0.5
1	49.5	44.4	38.3	25.2	8.58
2	74.7	72.2	68.8	56.2	25.0
3	87.4	86.1	84.4	76.6	41.8
4	93.7	93.1	92.2	87.9	56.2
5	96.8	96.5	96.1	93.8	67.8
6	98.4	98.3	98.0	96.9	76.6
7	99.2	99.1	99.0	98.4	83.1
8	99.6	99.6	99.5	99.2	87.9
9	99.8	99.8	99.8	99.6	91.4
10	99.9	99.9	99.9	99.8	93.8
	100.0	100.0	100.0	100.0	100.0

1 Area 0→n = $\int_0^n C_1\, dn = 100\left[1-\left(\frac{\gamma \cdot 2^{-n} - 2^{-\gamma n}}{\gamma - 1}\right)\right]$

2 $C = 69.3 \left[\frac{\gamma}{\gamma-1}\right]\left[2^{-n} - 2^{-\gamma n}\right]$

Table XII. Apparent bioavailabilities based upon previous areas 0→n assuming γ = 100 is the standard

n	γ				
	100.0	10.0	5.0	2.0	0.5
1	100.0	89.7	77.4	50.5	17.3
2	100.0	96.7	92.1	75.2	33.5
3	100.0	98.5	96.6	87.6	47.8
4	100.0	99.4	98.4	93.8	60.0
5	100.0	99.7	99.3	96.9	70.0
6	100.0	99.9	99.6	98.5	77.8
7	100.0	99.9	99.8	99.2	83.8
8	100.0	100.0	99.9	99.6	88.3
9	100.0	100.0	100.0	99.8	91.6
10	100.0	100.0	100.0	99.9	93.9
∞	100.0	100.0	100.0	100.0	100.0

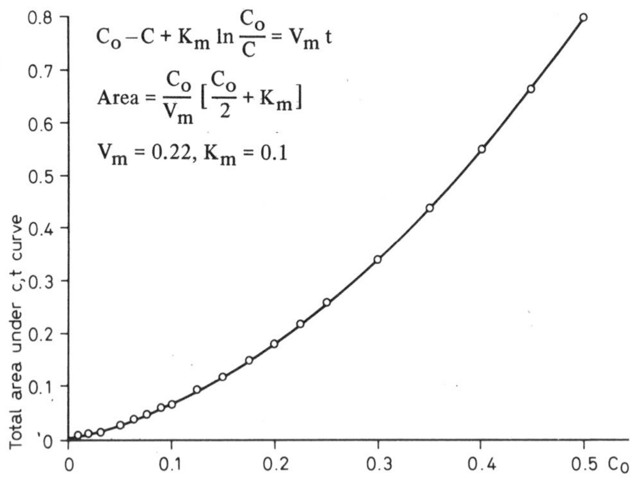

C_o	Saturation at C_o, %	Area	True availability of 'poor product', %	Estimated availability of 'poor product', %
1.0	90.9	2.7273	–	–
0.5	83.3	0.7958	50	29.2
0.25	71.4	0.2557	50	32.1
0.125	55.6	0.09233	50	36.1
0.0625	38.5	0.03729	50	40.4
0.03125	23.8	0.01642	50	44.0
0.015625	13.5	0.007657	50	46.6
0.0078125	7.25	0.003690	50	48.2
0.00390625	3.76	0.001810	50	49.1
0.001953125	1.92	0.0008965	50	49.5

Fig. 4. Total area versus dose curve.

Tables XI and XII illustrate the importance of measuring blood levels over a long enough time span. Blood levels should be measured at least over two and preferably over three elimination half-lives. If not, the area method is really invalid! Table XI shows areas calculated for the simple model shown in table X over various numbers of half-lives (n) and for various values of the ratio, γ = (rate constant for absorption/rate constant for elimination). Table XII summarizes apparent bioavailabilities based on the areas listed in table XI. Note that when the area is measured over only one half-life, the error is very large! Despite

Classical

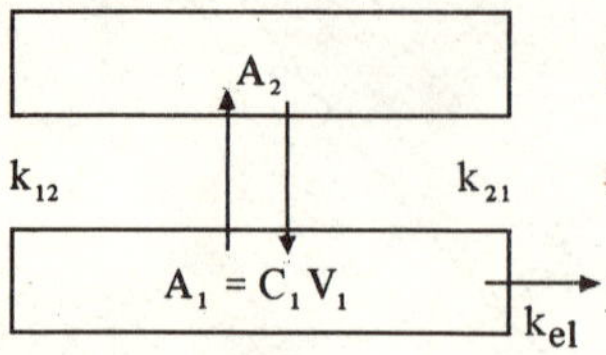

$$(dC_1/dt) = -(k_{12} + k_{el})C_1 + k_{21}C_2$$

$$(dC_2/dt) = k_{12}C_1 - k_{21}C_2$$

where $C_2 = A_2/V_1$ and $C_O = D/V_1$

Semi-classical

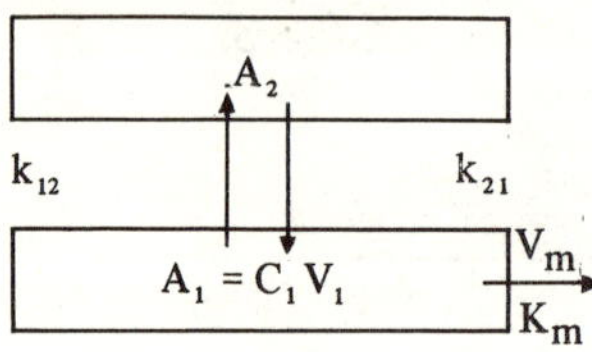

$$(dC_1/dt) = -k_{12}C_1 - (V_mC/(K_m + C)) + k_{21}C_2$$

$$(dC_2/dt) = k_{12}C_1 - k_{21}C_2$$

where $C_2 = A_2/V_1$ and $C_O = D/V_1$

Modern and future

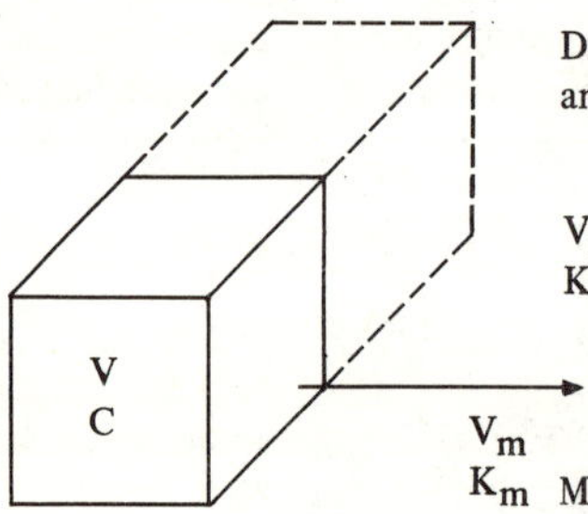

Drug in blood and o.f.d. (V.C.) + Tissue (A′–T′) $\underset{k_2}{\overset{k_1}{\rightleftharpoons}}$ Tissue-bound drug (T′)

$\downarrow$ V_m, K_m

Metabolites in blood
+
Unchanged drug in urine

If tissue and blood concentrations available use:

$$(dC/dt) = -k_1(A'-T')C - (V_mC/(K_m + C)) + (k_2/V)T'$$
$$(dT'/dt) = k_1V(A'-T')C - k_2T'$$

If only blood concentrations after several doses available use:

$$(dC/dt) = -k_1V(A-T)C - (V_mC/(K_m + C)) + k_2T$$
$$(dT/dt) = k_1V(A-T)C - k_2T$$
where $A = A'/V$ and $T = T'/V$

Fig. 5. Models.

this well-known fact, papers are still being published where the area is calculated over only one, or even less than one, elimination half-life.

Figure 4 illustrates another serious pitfall. Bioavailability studies must be performed at *low doses* of drug so that the enzymes metabolizing the drug, or the kidney transport mechanism, are all less than about 15 % saturated at all times following all dosage forms. In the region of 0–15 % saturation, the total area versus dose curve is reasonably linear, and the error in the bioavailability estimate for a poor product – which is actually only 50 % availability – is not great, as shown by the figures corresponding to 13.5 % saturation and below. If the blood levels go high enough that the enzymes become more than 15 % saturated, then the error increases very rapidly with increasing percent saturation as figure 4 shows. This is one reason my group spend so much time trying to get very specific and very sensitive assays for drugs in blood and urine.

Lastly, figure 5 summarizes what I would like to call classical, semi-classical, and modern or future pharmacokinetic models in much the same way as one classifies music. All of these types of models are being used today. They fit different situations and experimental conditions. We will show in the next 2 years or so, however, that if you wish to fit, and adequately explain, data collected following administration of several different doses of a drug, then you must use a model such as shown at the bottom of figure 5. This type of model includes both *saturable* tissue binding and *saturable* elimination kinetics of the *Michaelis-Menten* type. We have been fortunate that the classical models have worked as well as they have, and, this is mainly due to the fact that they have been applied to data collected following administration of relatively low doses of drug, or to only one dose of drug. Once you start looking at blood levels measured after several different doses of drug, you realize how inadequate the classical models really are. The ideas for the new models were pioneered by *Lundquist and Wolthers* (6), *Dedrick and Bischoff* (7), and *Levy et al.* (8).

Glossary of Symbols

A = general symbol for area under concentration curve (equivalent to No. 2 or No. 3).

Area $0\rightarrow\infty = \int_0^\infty C(t)dt$ = area under concentration curve from zero to infinite time after a single dose.

Area $0\rightarrow\tau = \int_{t_1}^{t_2} C_\infty(t)dt$ = area under concentration curve within a dosage interval ($\tau = t_2 - t_1$) at the equilibrium state.

A_{oral} = area under concentration curve after oral administration.
$A_{i.v.}$ = area under concentration curve after rapid intravenous administration.
A_u^∞ = amount of unchanged drug excreted in the urine in infinite time after a single dose.

$(\bar{A}_u^\infty)_A$ = average amount of unchanged drug excreted in the urine in infinite time after a single dose as treatment A.

$(A_u)_0^\tau$ = amount of unchanged drug excreted in the urine during a dosage interval at the equilibrium state.

$[\bar{A}_u^\infty]_0^\tau$ = average amount of unchanged drug excreted in the urine during a dosage interval at the equilibrium state.

$(A/V_1)_{tn}$ = amount of drug absorbed in time tn divided by the volume V_1 of the two-compartment open model.

$[A_u + M_u]_0^\infty$ = total amount of unchanged drug and all metabolites excreted in the urine in infinite time after a single dose of drug.

$[A_u + M_u]_0^\tau$ = total amount of unchanged drug and all metabolites excreted in the urine during a dosage interval at the equilibrium state.

$\beta = -\left[\frac{d \ln C_1}{dt}\right]_{t\to\infty}$ = rate parameter observed from *terminal* 'blood' concentration data when $\ln C_1$ plotted *versus* time.

Also $\beta = \frac{1}{2}\left[(k_{12} + k_{21} + k_{el}) - \sqrt{(k_{12} + k_{21} + k_{el})^2 - 4\, k_{21} k_{el}}\,\right]$

C = concentration of unchanged drug in whole blood, serum or plasma at time t after a single dose.

C_∞ = concentration of unchanged drug in whole blood, serum, or plasma at time t after dosing at the equilibrium state.

C_1 = concentration of unchanged drug in the inner (No. 1) compartment at time t of the two-compartment open model.

$C_t = A_t/V_1$ = the amount of drug in the outer (No. 2) compartment of time t of the two-compartment open model divided by the volume, V_1, of the inner (No. 1) compartment.

D = the administered dose of drug (mass units).

$\bar{D}_A$ = the average administered dose obtained by assaying sufficient individual dosage units.

f = the fraction of the unchanged drug reaching the circulation which is ultimately excreted in the urine.

f_{mi} = the fraction of metabolite i which is formed in the body which is ultimately excreted in the urine.

F = the fraction of the administered dose which is absorbed (i.e. reaches the general circulation).

k_d = the urinary excretion rate constant for unchanged drug.

k_{fi} (i = 1,2,...n) = the formation rate constant for metabolite i.

k_{12} = the first order rate constant for transfer from compartment No. 1 to compartment No. 2 of the two-compartment open model.

k_{21} = the first order rate constant for transfer from compartment No. 2 to compartment No. 1 of the two-compartment open model.

k_{el} = the first order rate constant for overall elimination from compartment No. 1 of the two-compartment open model.

K = the first order elimination rate constant of the one-compartment open model.

k = the first order absorption rate constant of the one-compartment open model with first order absorption.

M_{ui}^∞ = the amount of metabolite i excreted in the urine in infinite time after a single dose of drug.

$[M_{ui}]_0^\tau$ = the amount of metabolite i excreted in the urine in a dosage interval at the equilibrium state.

$(\overline{M}_u^\infty)_A$ = the average amount of a specific metabolite excreted in the urine in infinite time following treatment 'A'.

r^2 = the coefficient of determination of a regression = $(\Sigma obs^2 - \Sigma dev^2)/\Sigma obs^2$

V = the apparent volume of distribution of the one-compartment open model.

V_1 = the volume of the inner (No. 1) compartment of the two-compartment open model.

$$V_{d\ area} = V_1 \left(\frac{k_{el}}{\beta}\right) = V_1 \left(\frac{\alpha}{k_{21}}\right)$$

W = body weight.

References

1 *Wagner, J.G.:* Biopharmaceutics and relevant pharmacokinetics. Drug intelligence publications, chap. 24, p. 166 (Hamilton Press, Hamilton 1971).

2 *Manninen, V.; Melin, J., and Härtel, G.:* Lancet, p. 934 (1971).

3 *Morris, C.:* R_X: brand or generic? Your decision may be important in a malpractice defense. Private Practice, p. 39 (1971).

4 *Wagner, J.G.:* J. pharm. Sci. *56:* 652 (1967).

5 *Loo, J.C.K. and Riegelman, S.:* J. pharm. Sci. *57:* 918 (1968).

6 *Lundquist, F. and Wolthers, H.:* Acta pharmacol. toxicol. *14:* 265 (1958).

7 *Dedrick, R.L. and Bischoff, K.B.:* Chem. Engng Prog. Symp. Ser. *64:* 32 (1968).

8 *Levy, G.; Vogel, A.W., and Amsel, L.P.:* J. pharm. Sci. *58:* 503 (1969).

Author's address: Prof. *John G. Wagner,* Pharmacy Service, University Hospital, The University of Michigan, *Ann Arbor, MI 48104* (USA)

Pharmacology *8:* 118–141 (1972)

Physiological and Pharmacokinetic Complexities in Bioavailability Testing[1]

Sidney Riegelman

Department of Pharmacy and Pharmaceutical Chemistry, University of California, School of Pharmacy, San Francisco, Calif.

In spite of the number of speakers that preceded this presentation, it is important to define bioavailability as viewed by this author. Bioavailability is a term used to indicate measurement of both the relative extent and rate at which an administered dose reaches the general circulation. In the context of this definition, the general circulation refers to the arterial and venous blood which carry the drug to the tissues, excepting the hepatic portal blood during the absorptive phase. Note that this definition includes the rate of bioavailability in addition to the extent of bioavailability. The rate at which a drug reaches the fluids of distribution controls the onset, the intensity and possibly the duration of pharmacological effect. It is, therefore, equally important to the evaluation of biological performance of a drug product as is the measurement of the extent of availability. There is, however, a great deal of ambiguity when one refers to the degree of absorption rather than the degree or extent of bioavailability. This is due to the fact that a portion of the drug may be absorbed into the blood stream, but during its transit through the gut wall and during its first pass through the liver, significant amounts of the drug may be converted to the biologically inactive form. This is referred to as the so-called 'first-pass effect'. There is also a confusion and ambiguity when one uses the term 'rate of absorption'. *Portmann* (1) recently proposed that the rate at which the drug becomes available to the blood be referred to as the rate of availability and the constant evaluated from the analysis of these data be referred to as the availability rate constant.

It is extremely important to realize no matter how simple it appears, all methods of data treatment to evaluate bioavailability of drug products are based on certain assumptions intrinsic in the pharmacokinetic treatment. Models are a way of visualizing the processes of pharmacokinetic events that take place in the

1 Supported in part by grant NIGMS 16496 from the National Institutes of Health, US Public Health Service, Bethesda, Md., USA.

subject under the specific conditions of the test. Models are not fixed, but change with the time, type of information one is attempting to obtain, the conditions of the test and the state of the subject. The bioavailability one calculates for a given formulation of product depends on many factors but in particular the final answer depends on whether the assumptions are valid in a particular application. The method and set of assumptions may be valid for the drug substance under a given set of conditions, yet they may be invalid when applied to a different set of conditions. Most models used in bioavailability analysis are built upon the assumption that factors controlling the rates of bioavailability, metabolism, distribution and excretion all can be appropriately described by first-order processes; and, therefore, that resultant models can be treated as linear systems. The purpose of this paper is to point out many factors that can possibly play a critical role in modifying the relative rate and amount of drug which can reach the site of action; and, therefore, influence the onset, intensity and duration of clinical response.

Fortunately, most drugs appear to distribute in the body, to be metabolized and excreted by first-order processes. However, there are many factors which can influence the process of absorption and cause it to be nonlinear in character. When attempting to define the rate of availability of a drug in the blood it has been frequently assumed that the overall process follows first-order kinetics. Drugs showing extremely rapid *in vitro* dissolution taken on an empty stomach may well appear to be adequately fitted by assuming that the rate of availability follows first-order kinetics. However, this is probably an untenable assumption for less soluble compounds and for many drug products when taken with food or when lying down. Even the rapidly dissolving product can be affected by dosage form characteristics (this will be discussed below). On the other hand, there is a growing list of drugs found to be nonlinear in their disposition processes. These often take place only under special clinical circumstances. Some of these abnormal situations can directly influence the relative rate and extent of bioavailability. Others that may not actively affect the bioavailability can appear to do so simply because they result in a change in the drug disposition model. What is more important, they can cause a significant change in the clinical response.

Initial bioavailability studies almost invariably are undertaken under ideal and reproducible conditions for obtaining maximum absorption of the drug product. It is usually administered to healthy, ambulatory subjects with a relatively large volume of water after overnight fasting. However, it is virtually impossible on the usual dosage regimen to take all doses of a drug product under the ideal conditions noted above. Therefore, at least some of the doses are exposed to conditions which cause irregular and incomplete absorption and may induce changes with the rate and degree of metabolism and/or drug excretion.

To be bioavailable, a drug substance must be in solution and must reach the site of absorption in a chemical form which is capable of being absorbed.

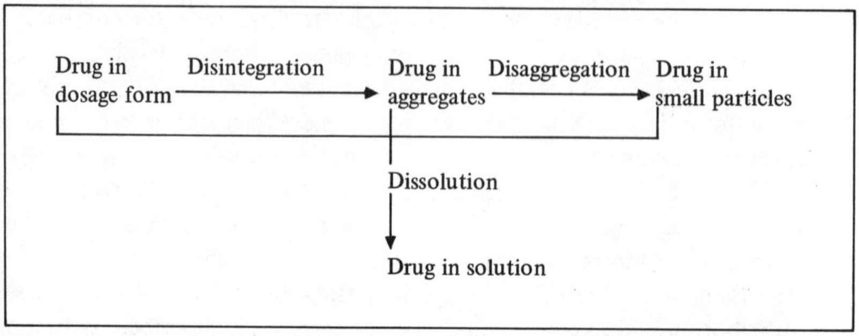

Fig. 1. Schematic representation of the disintegration, disaggregation and dissolution processes during the release of a drug from a tablet.

Figure 1 is a diagrammatic representation of the processes taking place when a solid dosage form undergoes dissolution. The intrinsic properties of the drug substance, the stirring rate and the characteristics of the dissolution fluids, of course, play important roles in this process. Many factors involved in the physical state and methods of combining the active components and excipients during the manufacturing of the dosage form cause marked changes in rate of disintegration and dispersion of the granules into the individual particles of drug substance. These processes cause a change in the rate at which the surface becomes available for dissolution. Since surface is gained – then lost – during this dissolution process, the overall data cannot be expected to behave as a simple first-order process. The processes of generation and loss of surface can be conceived to be more analogous to a probability function. This was pointed out by *Wagner* (2) who showed that almost all the existing data on drug *in vitro* release can be linearized, by plotting on probability paper, the percent dissolved against the time or log time.

In vivo this overall drug release process takes place in the presence of mucous and food. Either one can reduce the rate of water transfer into the dosage form and the diffusion properties of the drug molecule away from the surface. The gastrointestinal fluids, including bile, can interact with the drug molecules on the surface of the particle, in some cases solubilizing a drug and in other cases causing precipitation on the surface of the particle of a slowly dissolving form of the drug. The rate of dissolution will be modified by the intensity of peristalsis. The drug molecules also are exposed to bacteria and tissue enzymes which may metabolize a portion of the drug before it reaches the general circulation. These are examples of physiological factors which modify bioavailability. Figure 2 is a diagrammatic representation of some of the factors which can influence bioavailability. Table I is a listing of some of the dosage form factors and the physiological factors to be discussed below. Situations exist where such physiological factors will have a far greater effect on drug bioavail-

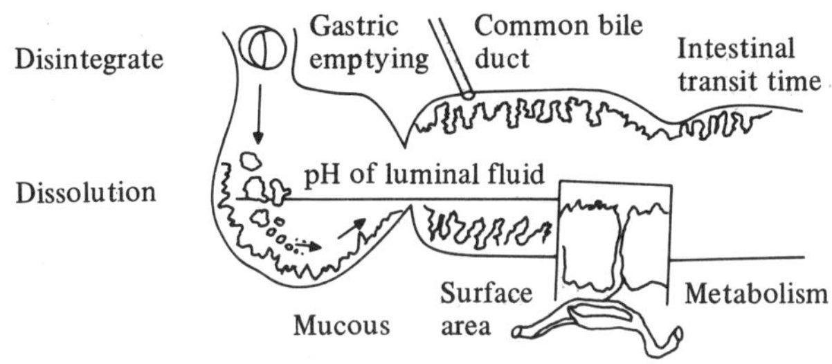

Fig. 2. Schematic of the stomach and intestines indicating some of the physiological factors which can influence the rate and extent of bioavailability.

ability than dosage form factors. These dosage form factors and physiological factors are interdependent, yet interacting phenomenon. It may be necessary to identify and separate the physiologic factors from the dosage form factors before meaningful evaluation of bioavailability of a drug product can be accomplished.

Let us return, however, to the gastrointestinal factors that may influence bioavailability. Figure 3 includes data obtained in the study of aspirin absorption from solution. Aspirin was administered to an individual test subject in solution in a sufficient volume of water wherein it could not precipitate on interaction with the body fluids. They were administered under a fasting state. The study was undertaken on test subjects sitting in a chair during the first $1^1/_2$ h of the study. Doses of 325 and 650 mg were administered under identical conditions and blood sampling was undertaken frequently during the absorption and post peak curve. These subjects had been previously studied intravenously with the 325 mg dose of aspirin. The data could therefore be analyzed by the so-called *Loo-Riegelman* method of evaluation of the rate of absorption. The data plotted in figure 3 represent the results of these studies (3). Note that the percent remaining to be absorbed is plotted on semilog function versus time. The lower portion of the curve indicates essentially the same half-life for absorption of the drug in each experiment. However, there appears to be a variation among the studies as to the time period before the system becomes log linear in character. One can explain these differences as possibly being due to differences in stomach emptying. We must conclude, therefore, that stomach emptying is complex and requires one to include time lags in analyzing absorption data. Additional experiments were done on dogs, operated so that their stomach was severed at the cardiac and pyloric ends (4). The esophagus was then attached directly to the duodenum. The stomach was then isolated and attached to a *Thomas* cannula so that the drug solution could be instilled into the stomach. Studies were done on the absorption of aspirin in solution as well as with other drugs. In every instance when solutions were administered to the dog through his esophagus di-

Table I.

Dosage form factors	Physiological factors
Physical properties of drug	Properties of luminal fluids
Water solubility	Hydrogen ion concentration
Lipid solubility	Mucous interaction
Partition coefficient	Complexing components
pKa	Surface activity
	Bile interaction
Properties of dosage form	
Disintegration time	Factors effecting GI transit
Dissolution rate	Gastric emptying
Surface area of particles	Food effects
Crystal size	Bed rest
Polymorphic form	Motility
Solvates	Enterohepatic cycling
Salt form	
Excipients	Factors of site of absorption
	Surface area
Manufacturing variables	Permeability of barrier
Granulating process	Specialized transport
Lubricant concentration	Local blood flow
Compression pressure	Intestinal metabolism
Tablet coatings	
	Metabolic aspects
	Hepatic metabolism
	Enzyme levels
	Hepatic portal blood flow
	Drug binding proteins
	Extrahepatic metabolism
	Saturation phenomena
	Gut wall metabolism
	Kidney metabolism
	Distribution effects
	Plasma protein levels
	Obesity
	Disease states
	Achlorhydria
	Thyrotoxicosis
	Biliary atresia
	Congestive heart failure
	Pharmacological effect of drug
	Modification of blood flow
	Parasympatholytic activity

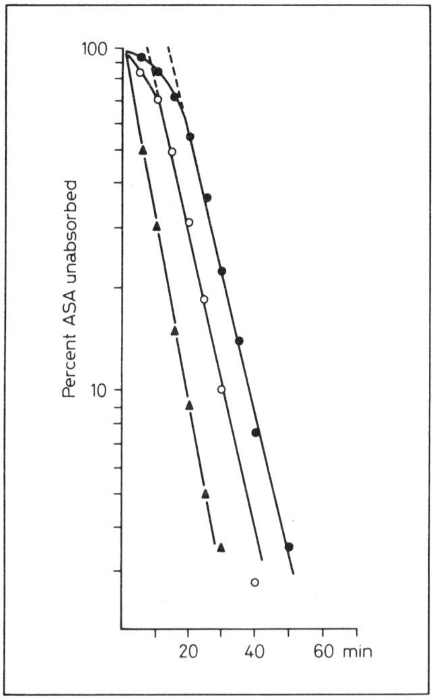

Fig. 3. Calculated data for the percent of aspirin unabsorbed from 325 (0,0) and 650 (0) mg doses of aspirin. The estimated half-lives for the terminal log linear portions are 6.8, 7 and 7.5 min, respectively. Data obtained from one test subject.

rectly into his intestines the resultant data indicated an extremely rapid absorption. The resultant blood curves almost superimposed on the i.v. data obtained for the same drug. However, when the drug was instilled into the stomach the rate of availability was extremely slow, usually less than one tenth that obtained when the drug directly reached the highly vascular intestine with a large surface for absorption.

When taken on an empty stomach with only a small amount of water, a solid dosage form may well dump into the thick layer of mucous which coats the stomach walls thereby impeding disintegration and dispersion of the aggregates. The components of the mucous can complex with some drugs; with others, the mucous blanket will cause an abnormal diffusion gradient to be generated. The extent of peristalsis and whether the subject is ambulatory or not will also contribute to how fast the drug product goes into solution and reaches the major absorbing sites in the intestines. Figure 5 is taken from the study of *Gianturco* (5) who investigated the stomach-emptying characteristics of the cat. The cat was fed 20 g of meat cut into lumps, then it was given milk mixed with barium sulfate, and represents an X-ray photograph of its stomach: (a) immediately

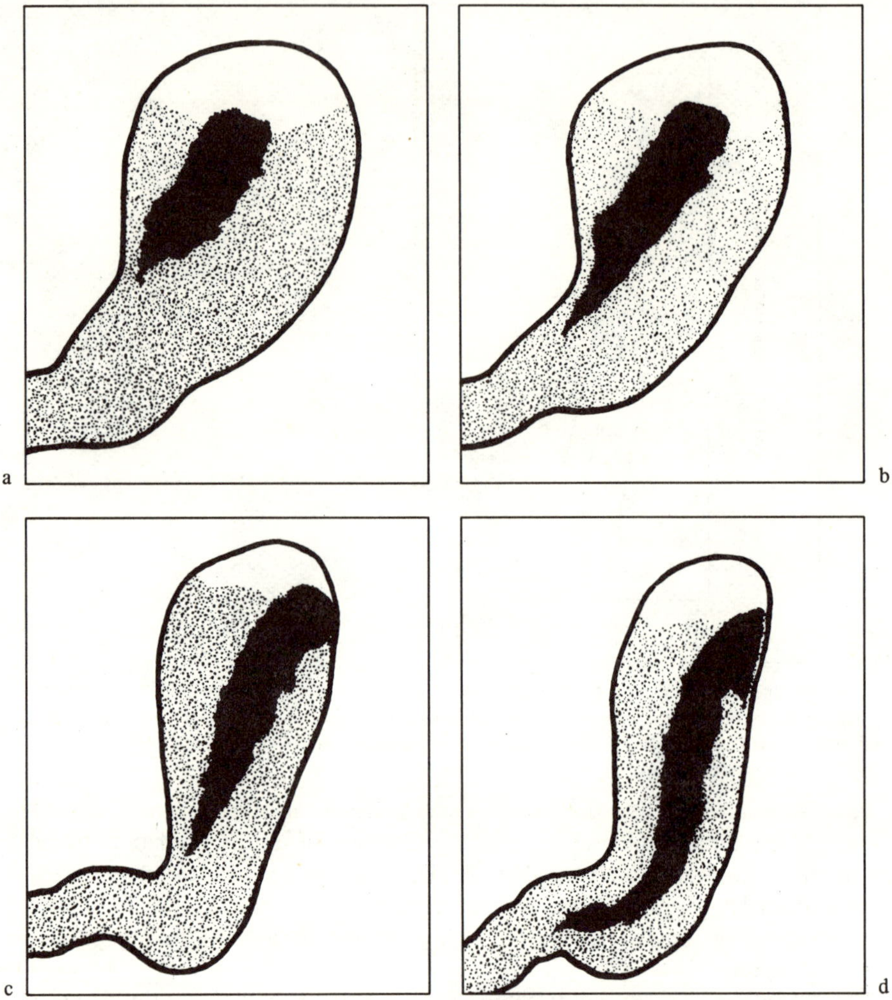

Fig. 4. Tracings of X-rays of the stomach of a young man immediately before (a) he ate 200 g of fried meatballs, the 50 g of meatballs mixed with powdered barium sulfate, and finally another 100 g of meatballs without contrast medium. (b) 10 min later; (c) 35 min later; (d) 65 min later (5).

after drinking the milk, (b) 10 min later, and (c) 20 min later. One can note the lumps in the body of the stomach which are outlined with barium, but most of the fluid has left the stomach and is in the small intestines. Thus, when taken with food, liquids empty out of the stomach rather more rapidly than solids. Slowly disintegrating tablets will be left behind within the solid matrix of food churning around within the stomach. Figure 4 is adapted from the work of *Niel-*

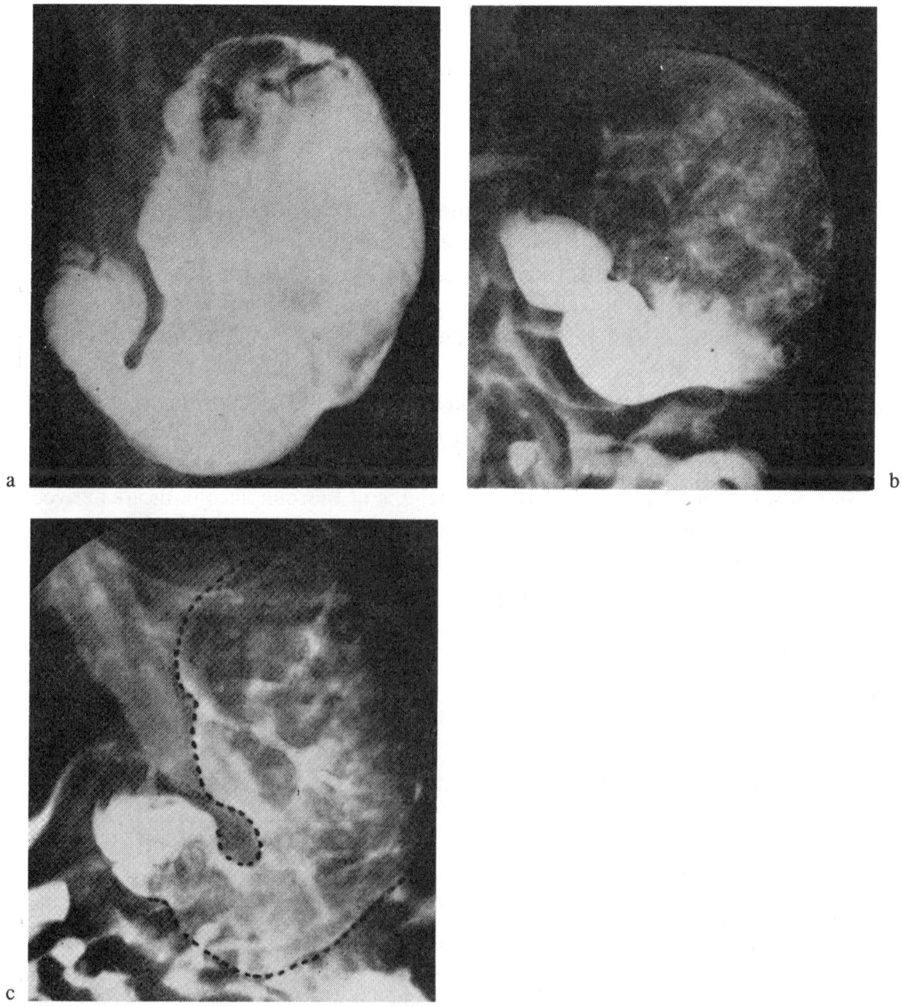

Fig. 5. X-rays of the stomach of a cat. The cat was fed 20 g of meat cut into lumps, was then given milk mixed with barium sulfate: (a) immediately after drinking milk; (b) 10 min later; (c) 20 min later (6).

sen and Christiansen (6). They were taken from X-rays of a man who had eaten 200 g of hamburger, was then administered 50 g of meatballs mixed with powdered barium sulfate; finally, another 100 g of hamburger without contrast medium. Figure 4a represents the stomach immediately after the meatballs with the contrast medium, figure 4b is 10 min later, figure 4c is 35 min later and figure 4d is 65 min later. Note that the solid radiopague material mixes with the food, is kept away from the absorbing surface, and churns around until it reaches the pyloric sphincter and ultimately is transported into the intestines.

The solid dosage forms containing poorly soluble weak acids can interact with the highly acidic fluids of the stomach to precipitate the slowly dissolving free-acid forms of the drugs. This is a common occurrence with drugs such as the anticoagulants, diphenylhydantoin, barbiturates, sulfa drugs and other weak acids. Even though the drugs are administered as a sodium salt upon reaction with the highly acid stomach fluids, the precipitated free-acid form will retard dispersion of the solid and, therefore, reduce the surface for dissolution. Even the gastric emptying can be affected since the solid mass will probably be emptied much more slowly than the hundreds of individual granules of which they are composed.

Cationic drugs administered as water-soluble salts can be equally affected. Sulfates and mucopolysaccharides can complex the drug molecules, and the components of the bile can also interact with the solid drug, or the drug molecules in solution. For example, the glycocholic or taurocholic anions are derived from strong acids, are of large molecular weight and relatively flat. They can interact with the drug cations, forming insoluble precipitates on the surface of the drug particles, impeding further dissolution. Many cationic drugs are frequently coated to prevent them from causing a bitter taste in the mouth during administration. At other times, they are coated since the tablet does not appear elegant unless it is covered with a colored coat. These dosage forms may be so formulated that the tablet mass will be left behind in the stomach, and may not disperse completely or dissolve prior to transport to the intestines. If the solid drug particles are transported to the intestines, there is good likelihood that some of them will be conjugated by bile anions, causing the precipitates discussed above. If dissolved, molecules of the drug may react differently with the concentrated bile components. They may interact to form ion pairs with the anions that in turn can be solubilized into the bile micelle. Exactly what happens to these different forms is difficult to define. It is important, however, to recognize that to merely test absorption of the drug on an empty stomach is illogical since one or more doses of these drug products are usually administered when the stomach is full of food. If the patient is bedridden, even administering the drug on an empty stomach can modify the dispersion of the drug into the granules and its ultimate dissolution and transit to the absorption site. This will also seriously affect the bioavailability. My personal view is that no dosage form has been adequately defined as to its bioavailability characteristics until studied under clinically logical situations of administration such as those indicated above.

Quinidine is a cationic drug whose clinical effect is directly related to the blood level. Blood levels of at least 3 mg/ml are required for cardiovascular activity and excesses of 5–7 mg/ml appear to result in undesirable side-effects. The free base of quinidine is quite insoluble. What is more important, its water

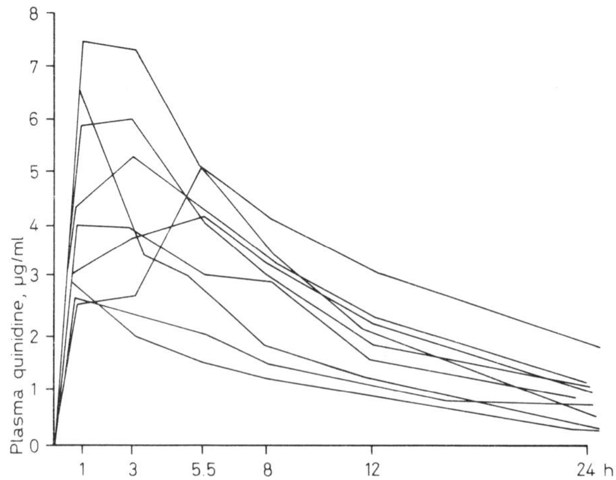

Fig. 6. Plasma levels after oral administration of 1 g of quinidine gluconate (7).

soluble forms interact with the conjugated bile anions to form an even more insoluble product. This drug is extremely affected by being administered with food. Once again, it is almost impossible to administer the dosage three times a day without interacting with at least one meal during the day. It is, therefore, important to develop a dosage form of the drug which will release the compound and make it available for dissolution before it reaches the intestinal tract. Figure 6 includes data obtained (7) after the administration of 1-gram doses of quinidine gluconate. Note the variability of the curves obtained from different subjects; even when administered on an empty stomach at least some of these problems are due to the interactions with the constituents of the gastrointestinal tract. When repeated with subjects who had eaten prior to taking the drug, the data show even less bioavailability and result in peaks which rarely reach the 3 mg/ml required to yield therapeutic response.

The data on the complexities of the availability of tetracycline hydrochloride have been discussed in *Barr*'s presentation. The data clearly indicate that the dissolution of tetracycline hydrochloride from dosage forms is pH dependent. If administered with food, or antacids, or when the patient is bedridden, the drug shows significant limitations in its bioavailability. At the last count in California, over 150 generic brands of tetracycline hydrochloride were under distribution. How many do not disperse properly in the presence of mucous, food, or on an empty stomach is not known. Tetracycline was introduced over 20 years ago. It is a tragedy that it has taken us 18 of these 20 years to appreciate the effects of dosage-form factors on its bioavailability.

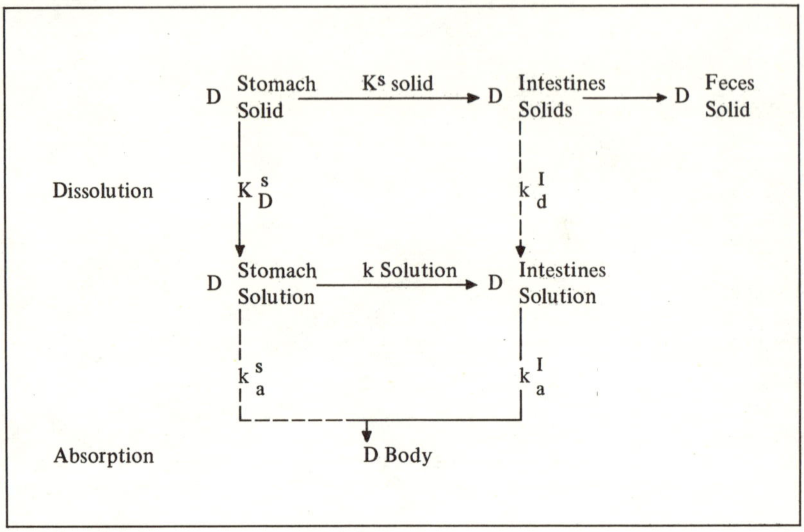

Fig. 7. Schematic representation of dissolution and stomach emptying, emphasizing how they may interact to modify the rate and extent of bioavailability.

Figure 7 is a schematic drawn originally by *Barr* (8) to represent the dissolution and absorption processes involved with tetracycline; however, this can be generalized to many drugs. The major route for ultimate absorption is the solid entering the stomach, hopefully going into solution in the stomach, and the solution being emptied into the intestines where absorption takes place. If, however, the solid empties into the intestines, a fraction of this may remain unabsorbed and may or may not be eliminated in the feces as unavailable drug. It certainly behooves us to define *in vitro* drug-release procedures to screen drugs such as tetracycline hydrochloride as soon as possible. I do not believe we can rest on the glib and unproven tenet that dosages of tetracycline hydrochloride are in excess of that which is needed for the full therapeutic effect, and, therefore, enough gets absorbed irrespective of these reactions. *Barr* has shown that when tetracycline is given with food or when the subject is bedridden the resultant blood levels show a correlation with the present *in vitro* tests (8). This data should be obtained for other drugs. Before leaving the topic of the factors which may cause the availability rate of a drug to be nonlinear in character, I would remind you that the only way one can fully analyze the data obtained from a blood study, under these circumstances, is to compare the data with that obtained after intravenous administration or under conditions where the rate of availability of the product to the general circulation is accurately defined. One

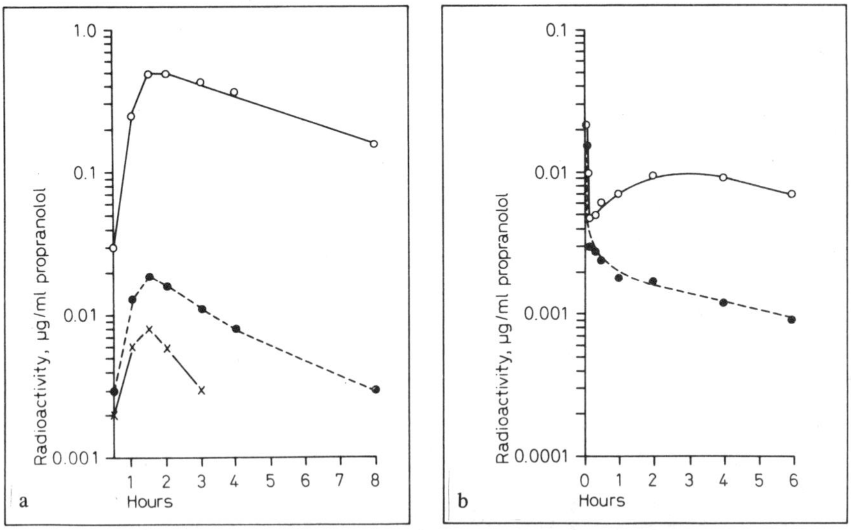

Fig. 8. Blood levels of propranolol, 4-hydroxypropranolol, and total plasma radioactivity following administration of propranolol either intravenously or orally: (a) after 40 mg given orally; (b) after 1 mg given intravenously. Total radioactivity (○); ^{14}C-propranolol (•); ^{14}C-4-hydroxypropranolol (X) (10).

can make a full study of the availability process for orally administered dosage forms by appropriate analysis of these data, for example, using the *Loo-Riegelman* method of analysis (9). The post peak curve obtained from these studies occasionally shows a change in slope which may or may not be due to prolonged absorption. This is due to the fact that a slow, but prolonged absorption of 5–20 % of the dose is sufficient to cause a significant change in this terminal log linear slope. If a drug is poorly soluble, and therefore dissolves slowly, it is possible that the absorption-rate process is the rate-limiting step. Under these conditions, the descending portion of the curve predominantly reflects the absorption phase. This has been referred to as the flip-flop model, since the up curve represents the disposition phase and the down curve the absorption process. After absorption ceases, the curve once again becomes parallel to the i.v. slope. Unfortunately, due to limitations of the assay, this may not be seen. Prolonged absorption phase may be desirable for some drugs and undesirable for others. Substances with prolonged absorption phases may show large variation in their dosage-form modified bioavailability. They may also be subject to changes in bioavailability due to physiological factors such as gut transit time, peristalsis, etc.

A generally inappreciated phenomena related to drug availability is the so-called first-pass effect. *Barr* has discussed the data he has obtained with the

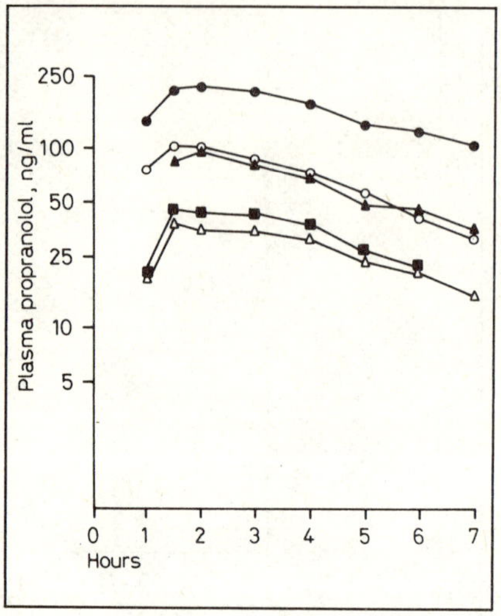

Fig. 9. Concentrations of propranolol in fasting subjects administered oral doses of 80 mg of propranolol (11).

salicylamide which is affected by the metabolism in the gut wall as well as during the initial pass through the liver. Since the intact molecule is presumed to be required for pharmacological activity, the rate and the extent to which the administered dose reaches the general circulation is important to such a drug. There are other examples. Propranolol is a well-known β-blocker which appears to show first-pass effects. Figure 8 is taken from the work of *Dollery et al.* (10) who administered 1 mg of the drug intravenously and 40 mg orally. Correcting for dose, based on area under the curves, the oral route leads to bioavailability. Also, the metabolite, 4-hydroxypropranol, an active β-blocker, is only detected when the drug is given orally. The lower curve on the right indicates the blood level of the intact drug after i.v. administration. The data of *Shand* (11) et al., illustrated in figure 9, complement *Dollery*'s findings. These data are after oral administration of 80 mg of propranolol to fasting subjects. Note this is a semilog plot and that peak blood levels range from 30 ng/ml to near 250 ng/ml. This almost 10-fold range of blood levels has a profound effect on the pharmacological activity of such a compound. If this drug was administered to subjects under conditions where absorptive phenomena modify its bioavailability, the subjects may show even larger changes when compared to the fasting state. Lidocaine, an amide containing local anesthetic, results in large variations of blood levels on oral administration (12). All the drugs mentioned are characterized by extensive hepatic metabolism and their clearances approach liver blood flow. As the half-life is a function of clearance and volume of distribution, it is possible for drugs

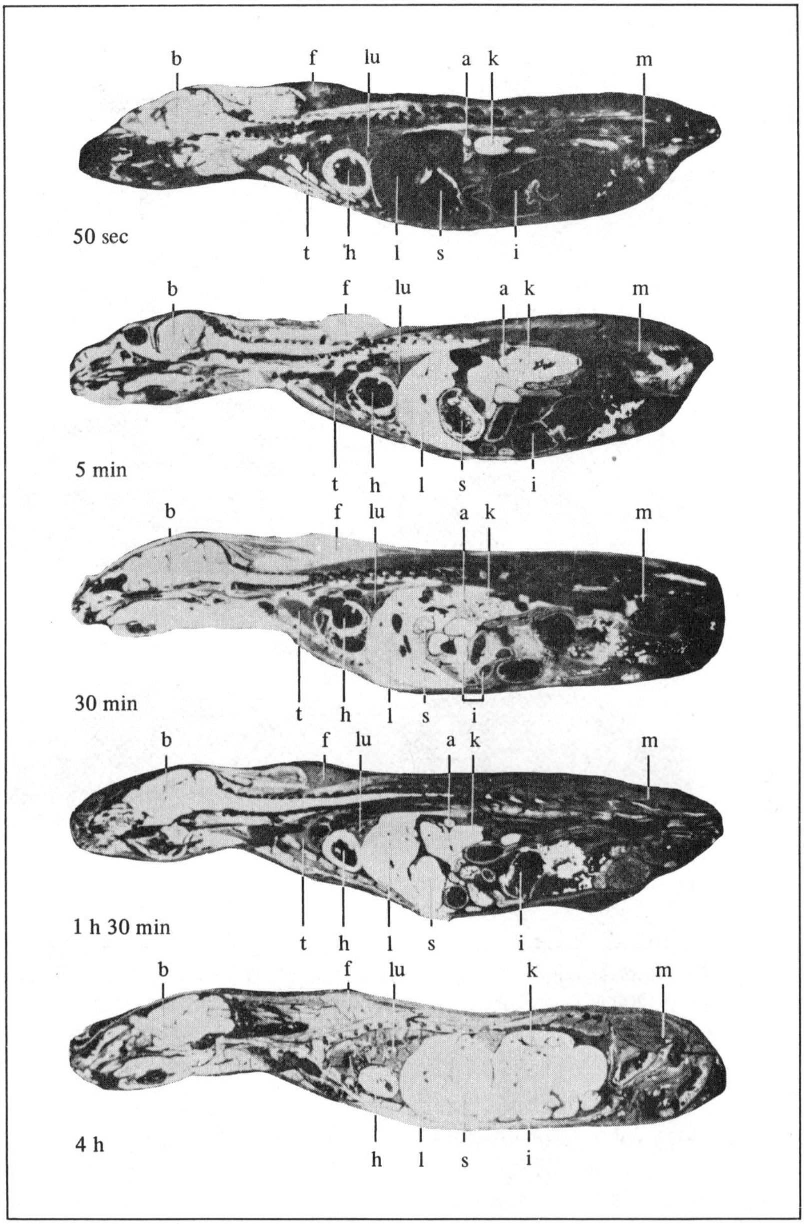

Fig. 10. Autoradiograms showing distribution of ^{14}C-diazepam and radioactive metabolites in mice after i.v. injection of 15 ng (200 μCi)/kg. White areas in autoradiograms correspond to high activity (15). b = Brain; f = fat; lu = lung; a = adrenal; k = kidney; m = muscle; t = thymus; h = heart; l = liver; s = stomach; i = intestine.

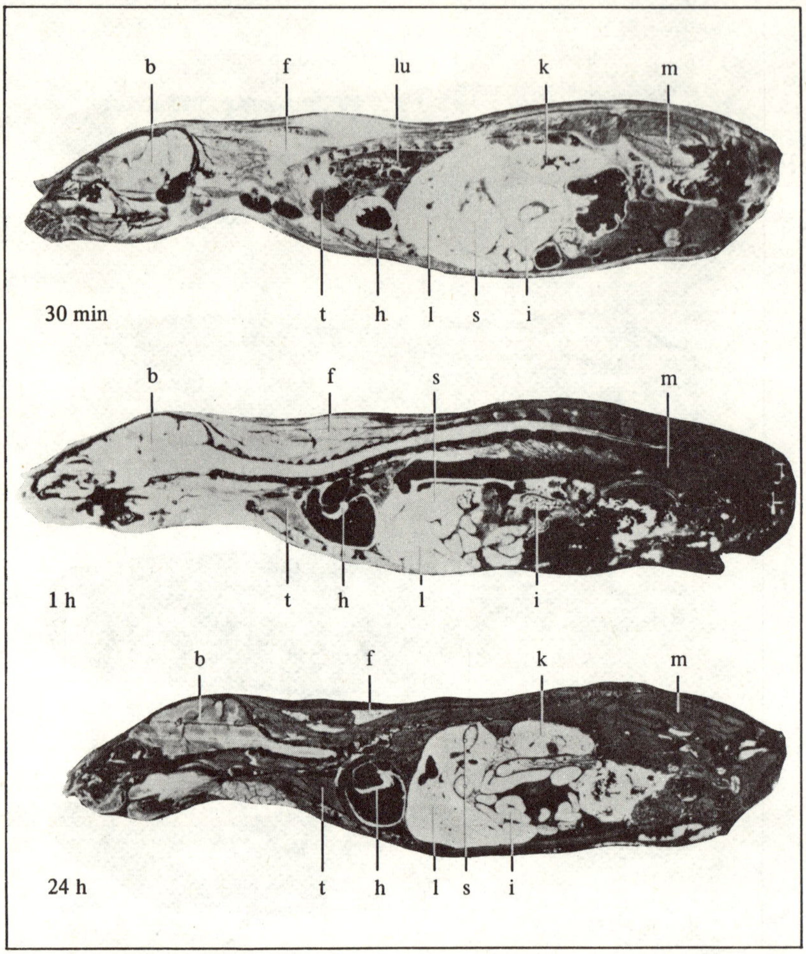

Fig. 11. Autoradiograms showing the distribution of ^{14}C-diazepam after oral administration of 30 ng (200 μCi)/kg. High concentration in the liver at 30 min (15). b = Brain; f = fat; lu = lung; a = adrenal; k = kidney; m = muscle; t = thymus; h = heart; l = liver; s = stomach; i = intestine.

with very large volumes of distribution to have long half-lives even though they are extensively cleared by the liver. When the clearance of a drug approaches hepatic flow it will be characterized by similarity in the disposition curve among subjects receiving the drug intravenously. While large differences in the oral availability will be anticipated as it is the difference between hepatic flow and clearance, minor differences between these quantitates will be magnified when given orally.

This first-pass effect is seen not only with drugs which have relatively short disposition half-lives, it has also been noted with compounds whose half-lives are greater, i.e. extending from 24 to 48 hours. Diazepam is a compound which shows this response as well as enterohepatic cycling. Figures 10 and 11 are the results of whole body autoradiography studies of *van der Kleijn* on diazepam administered to mice (13). The mice administered ^{14}C-labeled diazepam are killed, frozen and microtomed. The microtomed sections are exposed on X-ray film and the film developed so that the white portion on the pictures indicates the concentrations of the radioactive diazepam in the various tissues. Comparison of the concentration of the drug in the liver, stomach and gastrointestinal tract after i.v. and oral administration clearly indicates that there is a large amount of the radioactivity concentrating in the liver during the first pass. Human bile isolated from patients with bile fistulas has been observed to contain intact diazepam as well as its metabolites. This intact diazepam can undergo enterohepatic cycling as is shown in figure 12 where single doses of diazepam have been administered to subjects (13). Each of these curves show secondary peaks during the post-absorptive phase. Figure 13 illustrates the blood levels of diazepam after multiple dosing (13). It is to be noted that concentration of the

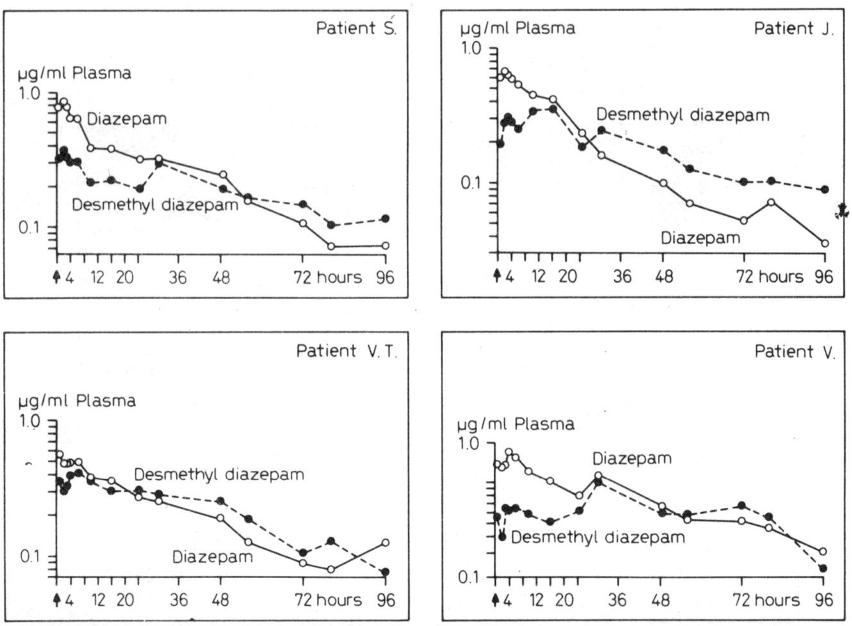

Fig. 12. Log concentration-time curves of diazepam and its major metabolites N-desmethyldiazepam after an initial dose of 30 mg. Note secondary peaks in curves after initial peaks probably due to enterohepatic cycling (15).

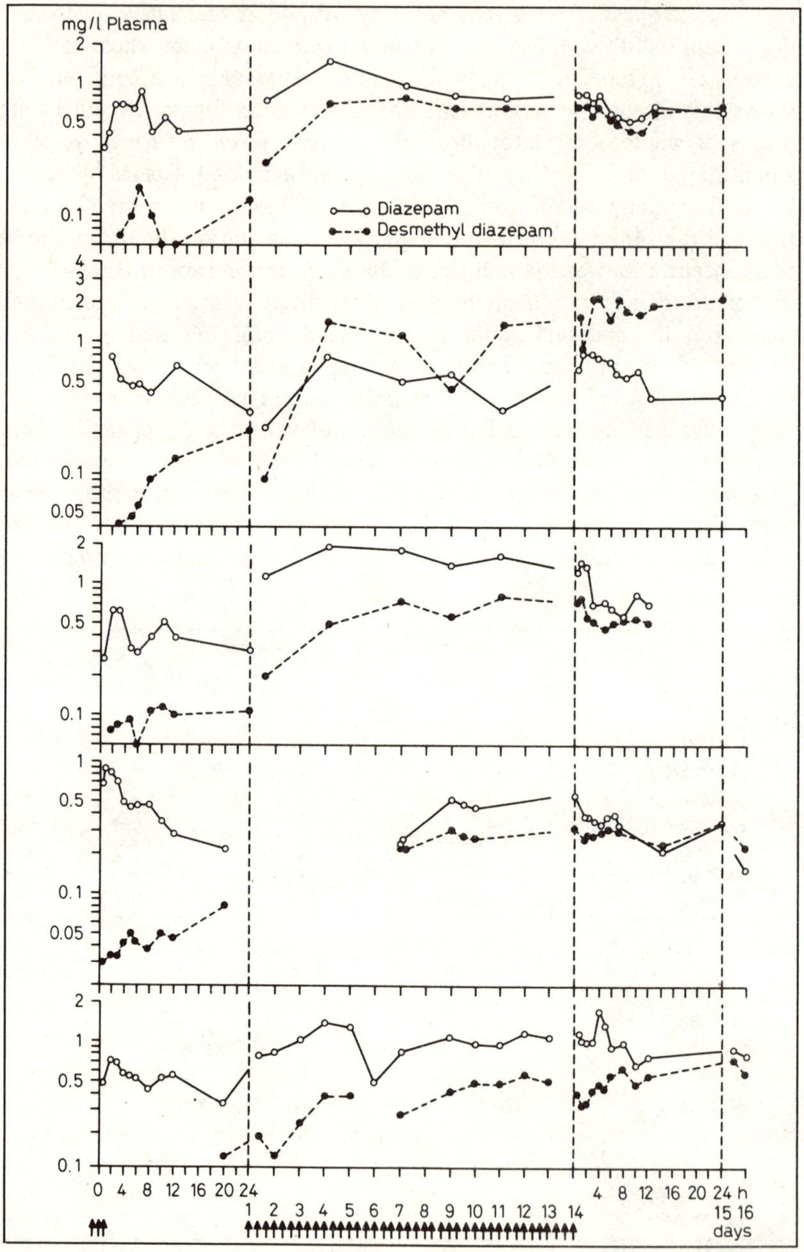

Fig. 13. Log concentration-time curves of diazepam and its major metabolites N-desmethyldiazepam during chronic treatment with 3 daily doses of 10 ng diazepam orally for 14 days (15).

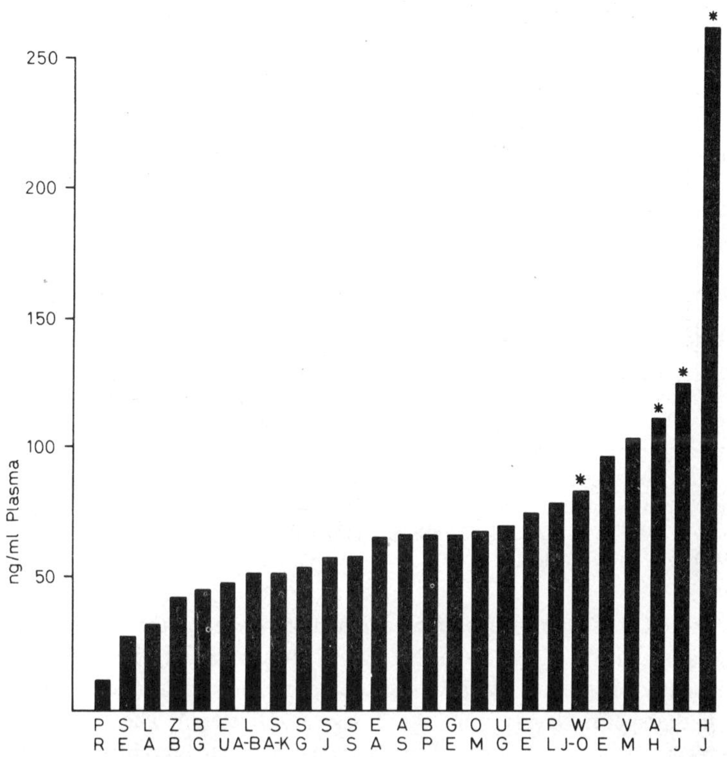

Fig. 14. Inter-individual differences in steady-state plasma concentrations of nortriptyline during daily oral dosage of 3 × 25 mg (16).

drug in the blood reaches a plateau on prolonged administration. The first-pass effects and subsequent enterohepatic cycling can somewhat be overemphasized in a drug such as diazepam. However, let us turn to nortriptyline and desmethylimipramine (DMI); both are tricyclic antidepressant compounds. Each has been found to show extensive differences in the plateau levels obtained when administered to subjects under identical dosing schedules. For example, figure 14 is from the data of *Alexanderson et al.* (15) who administered 250 mg of nortriptyline, until a plateau level was reached. The plateau level varies from approximately 30 to 260 ng/ml. *Hammer et al.* (15) obtained a similar set of data in studies on DMI. Part of this large variability can be ascribed to differing half-lives, part to differences in the volume of distribution. However, the literature data suggest that the clearance of these drugs (almost exclusively by the liver) is

15 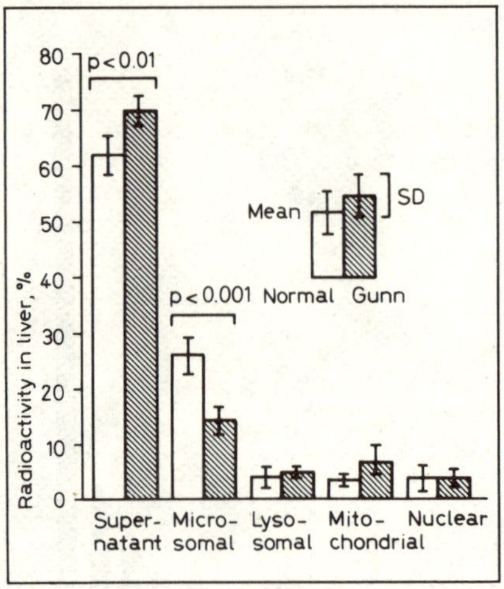

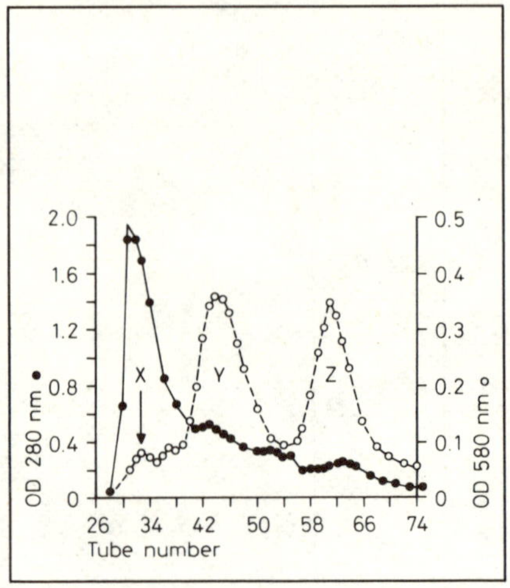 16

Fig. 15. Subcellular distribution of radiolabeled unconjugated bilirubin up to 60 min postadministration of ^{14}C-labeled bilirubin to normal and Gunn rats (18).

Fig. 16. The X, Y and Z sulfbromophthalein (BSP) binding protein fractions from 100,000 *g* rat liver supernatant (18).

higher and it is interesting to speculate that some of the observed variance is associated with a first-pass effect. Note that some of the subjects obtained sufficiently high blood levels to lead to undesirable side reactions. Others did not reach therapeutic levels from the dosage administered. The effect of food and other physiological or dosage form variables may also modify their bioavailability. Data will be given which supports the contention that this first-pass clearance by the liver is not linear in character and will therefore be concentration dependent. Thus, the rate at which the drug enters the hepatic portal vein will modify the amount of the intact drug which reaches the general circulation and exerts its therapeutic effect. Clearly, the metabolism kinetics of this drug vary from subject to subject, yet procedures can be devised for analysis at one or two data point times after the administration of a single dose of the drug, thereby allowing one to calculate the plateau level that would be reached upon continual administration of this amount of the drug. The dosage could then be adjusted appropriately to bring it into the therapeutic range. However, without adequate data of the influence of factors affecting the rate and extent of availability of the drug, the subject may vary from non-therapeutic to toxic levels.

When radioactive anions are administered to rats and their liver tissues are subsequently analyzed, it is found that the majority of the radioactivity is in the protein fraction (fig. 15). This protein fraction can be further subdivided by centrifugation and passage through molecular weight fractionating sephadex columns. The data shown in figure 16 are representative of the results obtained (16). The study

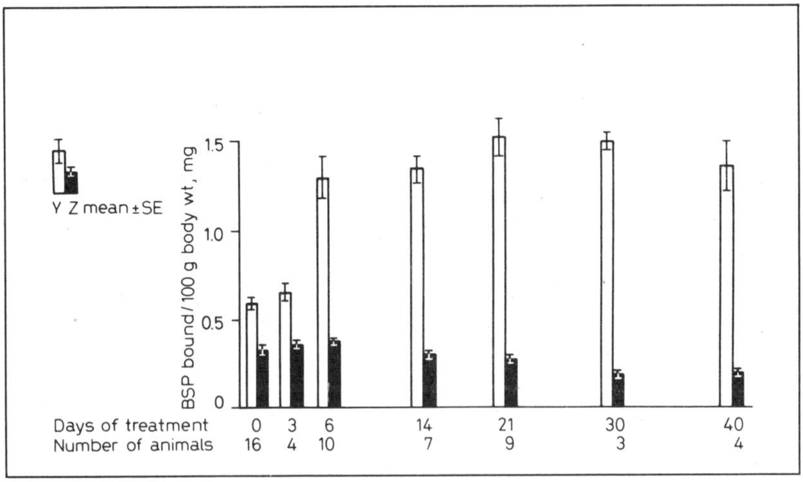

Fig. 17. Effect of daily phenobarbital administration (8 mg/100 g body weight) on Y and Z hepatic cytoplasmic proteins, as measured by BSP binding *in vitro*. Reproduced by permission of Proc. nat. Acad. Sci., Wash. (18).

was done using bromsulfonephthalein (BSP) as the tag. Each fraction eluting from the sephadex column was examined spectrophotometrically at 280 nm, which allows us to have a rough assessment of the quantity of protein material in the eluate, as well as 580 nm which is the maximum absorption wave length of BSP. It must be noted there are two extremely rich BSP-binding protein fractions, Y and Z. Phenobarbital, chlorinated hydrocarbons and other similar agents are frequently referred to as enzyme inducers; however, they also influence the amount of protein-binding fractions found in the liver. Figures 17 and 18 include data obtained through daily administration to rats of 10 mg of phenobarbital per 100 g of body weight (16). On continued treatment the Y-protein fraction increases markedly. There is also some increase of the Z-protein fraction. When animals pretreated with phenobarbital are administered BSP, the elimination rate constant increases roughly parallel with the increase in binding proteins (fig. 18). Fasting has the reverse effect. Thus, the binding capacity of the liver can be changed in status with many different types of treatment. Concomitant administration of other drugs can not only cause the liver metabolizing enzymes to change but modify the concentration of binding protein levels in the liver. In the absorptive phase where high concentration of drugs are transitting through the liver, it is likely that we enter into nonlinear kinetics due to this binding phenomenon. This is due to the fact that both the concentration of the drug and the binding protein must be considered in the equation. The rate at which a drug reaches the liver as well as a quantity of these two binding proteins will affect

18

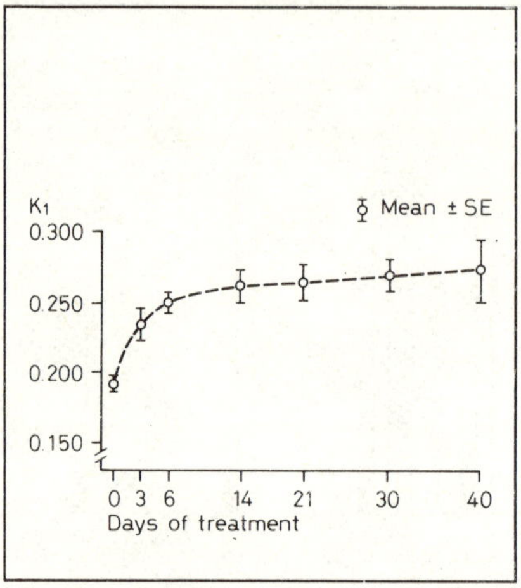

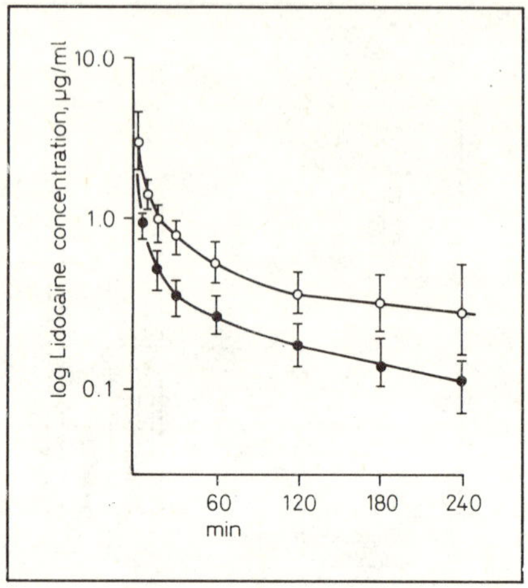

19

Fig. 18. Effect of daily phenobarbital administration (8 mg/100 g body weight) on K_1, the first-order rate constant for sulfobromophthalein removal from plasma. Reproduced by permission of Proc. nat. Acad. Sci., Wash. (18).

Fig. 19. Mean log concentration-time curves for lidocaine administered to normal healthy subjects (•), heart failure subjects (○).

the amount of drug reaching the systemic circulation. Similar proteins are likely to be found in the liver for cationic bound drugs.

It is also well recognized that the drug or some of its metabolites can directly or indirectly modify its rate of metabolism. This is seen with dicoumarol and with diphenylhydantoin when the blood level of the metabolites reach a concentration which may inhibit further metabolism or prolonged administration.

Not only does the liver binding and drug metabolizing capacity undergo potential saturation phenomena, but extrahepatic sites of metabolism show nonlinear phenomena as well. *Barr*'s data on metabolism of salicylamide are an example of saturation phenomena which appears to be taking place in the gut wall. Apparently the concentration of the gut metabolizing enzymes varies with the segment of the intestines studied. Therefore, in effect, the site of absorption of the drug will affect the degree of metabolism. The kidney is a very active site for drug metabolism. Data have developed which indicate that acetylation and glycine conjugation take place in animal and human kidneys to a degree that is competitive with and at times of larger magnitude than that found in the liver (17). The kidney metabolizing system has been shown to follow *M. Menton* kinetics. If the concentration of the drug transitting the organ is sufficiently high, the resultant data must be analyzed in accordance with *M. Menton* kinetics. What might not be immediately apparent is that these extrahepatic metabolism sites can affect the analysis of bioavailability. One should always keep in mind the statement made earlier that bioavailability analysis is model dependent. Since these changes markedly affect the model parameters, they must be taken into account to make an accurate bioavailability analysis. The rate constant of the model will change as well as the area under the plasma concentration-time curve. Unless these changes are properly defined, inappropriate conclusions may be drawn from the bioavailability analysis.

Additional conditions can affect the model parameters. We note marked differences in drug distribution in obesity. This has been particularly noted with diphenylhydantoin (18). It probably holds for other drugs. When the same mg/kg dose is administered to obese subjects, an increased distribution into the peripheral compartments was observed and a lower blood level resulted. Conditions which result in changes in the plasma proteins can affect drugs which are highly protein bound. Some are induced by hormones, including estrogens, progestogens, and thyroid hormones. These may modify both the albumin and globulin plasma protein levels. It is not often recognized that the albumin level can vary as much as 50 % from the average of 4 % w/v. Drugs which are highly protein bound will show different degrees of plasma binding. Changes in the distribution and metabolism will be seen at different concentrations of a total plasma level, which do not take into account the variation in the protein concentration. *Reidenberg et al.* (19) have shown that there is a difference in metabolism and disposition of diphenylhydantoin in the uremic state. We have seen the same results in seemingly normal subjects with reduced protein levels. Since highly protein-bound drugs are being administered to people under these conditions, it behooves us to define the elimination of such a drug under these states.

In addition to hyperthyroidism and uremia, there are other disease states which can markedly affect the distribution and the metabolism. Patients suffering from congestive heart failure will show marked differences in their distribution and metabolism of a certain drug. This is seen in figure 19, which includes the data from i.v. studies of lidocaine, done by *Thompson et al.* (20) within our University of California clinical pharmacology and pharmacokinetic groups. These are mean data from eight patients studied in each group and indicate a very large change in the volume of distribution within the central compartment as well as in the liver clearance. Note that the plasma clearance for lidocaine is more than 700 ml/min, which means that in one pass almost all of the total drug is removed by the liver. It is likely that this takes place both in the congestive state as well as in normal subjects. Yet the latter group have a mean clearance of only 310 ml/min. It is possible that with congestive heart failure, the subject simply has reduced blood flow to the liver. If drugs are administered orally to these subjects the clearance of the drugs in the hepatic-portal blood may differ and may be in the nonlinear kinetics region for a longer period of time. The

Table II. Pharmacokinetic data after the administration of lidocaine to normal and heart failure subjects

	Controls	Heart failure
$(t^1/_2)\beta$	108 min	115 min
V_p	0.53 l/kg	0.30 l/kg
metabolic clearance	10 ml/kg/min	6.3 ml/kg/min

amount of the drug reaching the central compartment will certainly change. Therefore, the therapeutic response to the drug can differ. (See also table II.)

Any factor-inducing changes in blood flow to various organs can make a difference in the metabolism and clearance of that organ. Thus, agents which induce changes in blood flow by their pharmacological action can cause changes in their clearance in the metabolizing and binding tissues. Some drugs can affect absorption by pharmacological action. For example, drugs with anti-spasmodic activity such as phenothiazines, parasympatholytics, antihistamines, and certain narcotic analgesics, can significantly suppress the peristaltic activity and thereby modify gastric emptying and gut transit. It was mentioned earlier by *Levy* that this resulted in at least one instance in the 5-fold increase in the magnitude of absorption of the drug. In other instances it will delay the stomach emptying and the onset of the activity as well as potentially modifying the amount absorbed.

Recommendations. The least ambiguous condition for initial bioavailability studies is in a fasted, ambulatory, healthy subject. I personally believe no drug has been adequately studied until we have examined the effect of food and bed rest on its bioavailability. Recognizing that certain physical chemical interactions can take place which can affect drug release, it is logical to attempt to mimic them *in vitro.* Exposure of the dosage form to carrageen (a sulfated gum) may mimic mucous effects. Exposure of the tablet or its granules to glycocholate and tauracholate anions can mimic the effect of bile on dissolution. Of course, changes in pH and stirring rate are additional variables to be examined.

Most drugs require dosing regimens and/or methods of treatment wherein one or more of the above discussed phenomena will be a complicating factor. Reexamination of the bioavailability during therapeutic trials and comparison of the results to normals (or after recovery of the same individual) may lead to evidence of marked changes in the bioavailability. One should then attempt to delineate the basis of the change. Model animal studies may afford evidence of what has taken place. While animals usually differ in the metabolism of a drug, they may afford an inexpensive monitor of bioavailability that is not easily reproduced by purely *in vitro* studies.

References

1 *Portman, G.:* Current concepts in pharmaceutical sciences; in *Swarbrick* Biopharmaceutics, chap. I (Lea & Febiger, Philadelphia 1970).
2 *Wagner, J.C.:* J. pharm. Sci. *58:* 1253 (1969).
3 *Han, S.K. and Riegelman, S.:* unpublished results.
4 *Harris, P.A. and Riegelman, S.:* unpublished results.
5 *Gianturco, C.:* Amer. J. Roentgenol. *31:* 735 (1931).
6 *Nielsen, N.A. and Christiansen, H.:* Acta radiol., Stockh. *13:* 678 (1932).
7 *Bellet, S.; Finkelstein, D., and Gilmore, H.:* Arch. intern. Med. *100:* 750 (1957).
8 *Barr, W.:* unpublished results.
9 *Loo, J.C.K. and Riegelman, S.:* J. pharm. Sci. *57:* 918 (1968).
10 *Dollery, C.T.; Davies, D.S., and Conolly, M.E.:* Ann. N.Y. Acad. Sci. *179:* 108 (1971).
11 *Shand, D.; McNicholls, G.E., and Oates, J.A.:* Clin. Pharmacol. Ther. *11:* 112 (1970).
12 *Rowland, M. et al.:* unpublished results.
13 *Kleijn, E. van der:* Pharmacokinetics of ataractic drugs (St. Catherine Press, Bruges 1969).
14 *Alexanderson, B. and Sjoqvist, F.:* Ann. N.Y. Acad. Sci. *179:* 739 (1971).
15 *Hammer, W. and Sjoqvist, F.:* Life Sci. *6:* 1895 (1967).
16 *Reyes, H.; Levi, A.J.; Levine, R.; Gatmaitan, Z., and Arias, I.M.:* Ann. N.Y. Acad. Sci. *179:* 520 (1971).
17 *Han, S.K. and Riegelman, S.:* J. pharm. Sci. (in press).
18 *Blum, R. and Levin, S.:* unpublished results.
19 *Reedenberg, M.N.; Cererlof, I.O.; Bahr, C. von; Borga, O., and Sjoqvist, F.:* New Engl. J. Med. *285:* 264 (1971).
20 *Thompson, P.D.; Rowland, M., and Melmon, K.L.:* Amer. Heart J. *82:* 417 (1971).

Author's address: Prof. Dr. *Sidney Riegelman,* University of California, School of Pharmacy, *San Francisco, CA 94122* (USA)

Pharmacology *8:* 142–147 (1972)

Newer Physicochemical Methods Useful in Bioavailability Studies

H.M. Fales

Laboratory of Chemistry, National Heart and Lung Institute, Bethesda, Md.

I wish to thank the members of this conference for introducing me to a most interesting and important problem. Furthermore, thanks should be expressed on behalf of those chemists and pharmacologists who are currently jobless, because it is my opinion that the solution to this problem will only be found by the expenditure of large amounts of money and effort by the pharmaceutical industry.

From an analytical viewpoint the problem seems to surround the measurement of small quantities of drugs, and secondarily their metabolites, in blood and urine. Analytical specificity is critical and a metabolite must be distinguished from the original drug. Furthermore, it seems to me that the methods must be comparatively straightforward since the analyses will be performed by physiologists and pharmacologists who do not wish to become involved with complicated apparatus. From the comments that have been made concerning statistical analysis it is also clear that it will be necessary to run a relatively large number of samples to obtain the reliability required by regulatory agencies.

In general, physical measurements depend either on the emission or absorption of radiation, the conduction of current, or the measurement of mass. Radioactivity has been, and will continue to be, extremely useful in the measurement of bioavailability, providing the experiment is designed with care. For example, if the main pathway of metabolism of a drug has been established as N-dealkylation, the drug could be analyzed accurately by direct measurement of the radioactivity of a simple extract of crude blood provided the drug was labeled differently, with tritium in the cleaved side chain and ^{14}C in the nucleus. Organic chemists are extremely skillful in selective synthesis of this sort, yet there are few examples of such approaches in the pharmacological literature. I suspect this is at least partly due to the appalling lack of communication between pharmacologists and most organic chemists. The only link between the two today seems to be the pharmacognist, whose main interest lies in the structures and taxonomy of natural products.

Tritium labeling by catalytic exchange is a synthetic procedure which is applicable to almost any aromatic or olefinic linkage and is simple enough to be carried out in the pharmacological laboratory, especially since the degree of labeling can be easily checked by conducting the experiment with deuterium and analyzing the product by nuclear magnetic resonance. This labeling technique is not to be confused with the highly destructive Wilzbach process which has given tritium labeling such a bad name in the protein field.

In radioimmunoassay methods, radioisotopes reach their peak utility, often justifying the labor spent in perfecting the assay. Whenever the subject of radioisotopes is brought up, the problem of radiation hazards is raised. It is my personal opinion that this objection is greatly overemphasized in the US. Surely the benefits from properly designed radioisotope experiments greatly outweigh the risks in most cases. Of course, it is indefensible to conduct such experiments solely for the purpose of evaluating a drug which represents a trivial modification, designed purely for competitive purposes.

Light absorption methods, i.e. color tests, ultraviolet and especially fluorescence analyses have been developed by the pharmacologist to a high degree of excellence and will undoubtedly continue to occupy an important place in his activities. Recently considerable improvements have been made in spectrophotometric devices allowing observation and accurate quantitation of samples under conditions of high dilution (low optical density), where there is a dense background (high optical density), and even where there is heavy scattering (turbid solutions). It seems likely that most of the conferees here are better versed in this subject than I and so I will not dwell on this aspect further.

Regarding the electric measurements, the method of cyclic voltammetry (a more modern version of polarographic analysis) seems to have enormous potential in analyzing drugs with oxidizable or reducible functional groups. In this method, two electrodes are immersed in the fluid to be analyzed, the voltage swept over a range of a few volts and the resulting current variation observed on an oscilloscope or a recorder. The polarity is then reversed and the voltage swept back to its original value. The time for this process is in the range of milliseconds to seconds. When millisecond times are used, the reducible (or oxidizable) species near the electrode is consumed by the process and the current falls forming an S-shaped peak of current versus voltage. If the reduced (or oxidized) product reacts with the medium, however, the subsequent reverse process may not be observed to proceed to the same point since there is less reduced material present. Such an effect is easily observed on the tracing and reflects reaction rates of the intermediates in a very precise manner. As such, the method may have a good deal of selectivity and is capable of quite precise quantitation, particularly when it is possible to analyze the data with a computer. The reduced species may be observed in an electron paramagnetic resonance device if the free radical produced has any stability. Furthermore it is a very precise way to measure many metal ions. Cadmium can be observed at 10^{-10} M concentrations if it is collected in amalgam at one electrode (stripping analysis).

Regarding the measurement of mass, the molecular weight of a compound is by itself a fairly characteristic identifying feature. If measurement is carried to significant accuracy (approximately three decimal places) it is even possible to obtain the formula of a compound – a very convincing argument as to its identity. The modern mass spectrometer allows such measurements to be made quite easily and further provides very conclusive identification by virtue of the characteristic fragmentation undergone by the molecular ion under electron bombardment. The method certainly provides the required sensitivity; it is even possible to speak of the measurement of numbers of molecules rather than fractions of moles. When combined with gas chromatography the utility of the mass spectrometer is enhanced manyfold, particularly in pharmacological and biochemical studies. In recent years it is true that it has been used mainly as a qualitative tool to provide evidence that a small peak observed in the gas chromatogram was positively due to the drug or metabolite in question. Its use as a quantitative tool has not been widespread and in the case of bioavailability studies, quantitation is clearly a key prerequisite. Still, there are many ways in which quantitation may be achieved. In the most obvious technique, a small quantity of drug which has been labeled with either ^{13}C, ^{15}N, or deuterium isotopes, is added to a known volume of blood or extract so as to provide an internal standard whose physical properties will be identical to those of the unknown, but whose mass will be easily differentiated from that of the unknown. The required labeled drugs are relatively simple to synthesize and of course provide no radiation hazards. Furthermore, the recently announced plans to increase the availability of ^{13}C and other heavy isotopes promises to stir up renewed interest in this area. However, it must be emphasized that sample handling is not particularly easy. Thus, the internal standard must be added to the extract of blood and the whole sample concentrated in a cup small enough to hold only a few microliters of the sample. The cup must then be placed into a high vacuum without losing the material and the sample heated just to the point that enough vapor is present to afford a satisfactory spectrum. If the heating is too rapid the sample may be lost before a spectrum can be scanned. If the heating is too slow, polymerization may occur – tyrosine is an example. The presence of impurities may occasionally be extremely troublesome when they have volatilities similar to the unknown. Gas chromatography can help enormously but it is no cure-all. The gas chromatographic column and support often has the annoying property of irreversibly adsorbing low levels of drugs as workers with chlorpromazine have noted.

An ancillary technique which has recently come into favor utilizes the mass spectrometer as a specific detector for the gas chromatograph. In this method the mass spectrometer is not scanned but the detector is set specifically at the molecular weight of an unknown so that the instrument responds only to compounds of this molecular weight. In this manner the mass spectrometer becomes relatively insensitive to all extraneous materials in the system and, because of the sensitivity of the electron multiplier detector, it is extremely sensitive for the given ion. Obviously, an intense or characteristic fragmentation peak of the drug might be used as well. However, increased reliability is obtained when not one, but two or even three ions resulting from fragmentation are monitored. This is achieved by rapidly switching the ion accelerating voltage to alternatively bring the several peaks into focus, a technique used for many years for the purpose of accurate mass measurement. Quite precise qualitative identification of the drug is possible at extremely low levels, even down to the picogram range in selected examples. However, precise quantitation at this level depends upon many factors such as amplifier gain, ion chamber condition, etc., that are not easy to maintain in constant day-in day-out operation of a mass spectrometer. Furthermore, the instrumentation is comparatively complex even in the case of the less expensive instruments available today, and the thought of performing 40 or 50 such analyses per day as may be required in bioavailability studies would not be kindly entertained by the average mass spectrometrist. An alternative which still does not satisfactorily answer precise quantitation problems is that of repeatedly scanning the gas chromatogram at fixed intervals (every few seconds) during the complete gas chromatogram. The numerous mass spectrograms are stored in a computer which then searches each for the desired ions. The output for each mass is then presented graphically and the result is simply an ion-specific gas chromatogram. Such plots can be presented for all masses pertinent to a given drug until sufficient confidence in its identity is obtained. In addition the complete mass spectrum at any time can be obtained from storage, but in many cases the drug in question may be hidden among the peaks due to an extraneous compound of the same retention time. Computer systems that will perform this operation are available in the $ 30,000–50,000 range. Of course, in this method some time is lost while ions foreign to the problem in question are being scanned by the mass spectrometer, although the time loss may be very small indeed if a very rapidly scanning mass spectrometer is employed. The advantage of such systems is that all data may be preserved, allowing the analyst to reinvestigate the problem from a different point of view after the analysis has been completed. Alternatively, it is even possible for the computer to drive the mass spectrometer to ions felt to be pertinent to the problem at hand, so that scanning time on insignificant ions is not wasted. Whether one technique or another is used is largely a matter of personal philosophy.

Specifically, regarding the mass spectrometry of drugs, our laboratory has recently been concerned with the method of 'chemical ionization'. In this system, originated by *M.S.B. Munson and F.H. Field,* an ion is formed from the compound, not by ionizing with an electron beam, but by allowing a proton from a previously ionized reagent gas to migrate from the reagent to the compound under analysis. The advantages of this system are that the energy introduced may be selected by the choice of reagent to be smaller than in electron impact, so that fragmentation of the molecule is minimized. In the case of many drugs and their metabolites only the molecular ion is observed (or more properly an ion at $(M + 1)^+$, i.e. $(M + H)^+$. The sensitivity of this method appears to be somewhat greater than electron impact for drugs although of course the characteristic fragmentation may be absent. However, in bioavailability studies it is ordinarily practical to run enough blank scans to ensure that the background is not providing an ion of the same mass and the overall simplification of the spectrum obtained in this mode is its most important feature. Of course, the regular electron impact mass spectrum may be obtained with such apparatus at any time merely by turning off the gas supply. It is my personal feeling that this technique should be extremely useful in studies of drugs and drug metabolism. However I must admit to mixed feelings regarding the application of mass spectrometric techniques to problems of bioavailability. I would like to encourage as many of you as I can to investigate the methods but at the same time I do not want to minimize the difficulties surrounding the operation of mass spectrometers and especially sample handling. Mass spectrometry is not a cure-all technique and will not yield useful results in such studies without the investment of considerable effort and time. For example, I know of no mass spectrometer produced today that will operate continuously without at least monthly maintenance of a relatively high order of sophistication. Furthermore, any attempt to depend upon the manufacturer's service facilities for this maintenance may be overly optimistic as any mass spectrometrist will sadly confirm. Instruments simply have not yet been built with the degree of reliability provided by scintillation counters and other laboratory instruments with which most of you are familiar.

What about other methods? Frankly, I do not see a great deal of hope from any other methods with which I am familiar. Infrared, even when coupled with gas chromatography using Fourier transform analysis, does not appear to possess the required sensitivity for such measurements. Nuclear magnetic resonance, again coupled with Fourier transform analysis, likewise does not possess the required sensitivity and the instrumentation is costly and complex. (It should be remembered that the highly touted Fourier transform methods only increase the sensitivity by a factor of ten at best.) Optical rotatory dispersion, except in the case of relatively pure samples of a few keto steroids is not nearly sensitive enough. The old standby, gas chromatography, will continue to be important and in this regard it is my own feeling that what is needed is the construction of a simple device to provide reasonably reliable identification of a gas chromatographic eluant. Perhaps a smaller, simpler, much less expensive gas chromatograph-mass spectrometer combination may be constructed some day. In very preliminary observations along this line we have set our resolution to be only ~ 10, i.e. m/e 10 is separated from m/e 11, and the resulting mass spectra of a GLC eluate is not much less valuable as a 'fingerprint' of a drug than one obtained with each peak resolved from its neighbor. The sensitivity is increased enormously since the apertures are wide open, but of course the individual peaks are smeared into each other and the molecular weight may be determined with an accuracy of only ± 1–2 atomic mass units. Such a device, employing the sensitivity of the electron multiplier detector at a cost of $ 3,000–5,000 would surely be a valuable tool to the gas chromatographer, particularly in bioavailability studies.

I hope that the enormous attendance at this meeting brings home to physical and analytical chemists as well as to manufacturers the fact that there is an immediate need for the design of truly automated methods for the reliable analysis of drugs in body fluids.

Author's address: Dr. *Henry M. Fales,* Chief, Laboratory of Chemistry, National Heart and Lung Institute, 9000 Rockville Pike, *Bethesda, MD 20014* (USA)

Pharmacology *8:* 148–152 (1972)

Panel Discussion

(Following Monday Session)

Question (audience): Is there a need for both intramuscular and subcutaneous bioavailability programs for aqueous preparations?

Response (Dr. Wagner): This answer applies to solutions not suspensions. Since many things can happen in the muscle, one cannot assume the same answer from i.m. as i.v. routes. Each route has to be checked. I have seen totally different results i.m., i.v. and subcutaneously with the same preparation.

Comment (Dr. Riegelman): I.v. may give trouble with a large dose of a water-soluble compound which may precipitate in the blood and result in an irregular disappearance curve.

Comment (Dr. Levy): The introduction of a drug at different rates by i.v. or other parenteral routes has an influence on compartmentalization and on the time course of drug action. I would caution approaching any bioavailability study with a set recipe. Any drug has problems of its own – put all of the information together and use proper judgment.

Comment (Dr. Riegelman): I am concerned about administering a drug to a patient who is initially in bed and then gets up – this has an influence on volume of distribution.

Question (Dr. Azarnoff): With regard to your statement (*Riegelman*'s) that one should study a drug over 7–10 half-lives, how long does a patient have to stay in bed?

Response (Dr. Wagner): That is why I propose using normal, ambulatory people. If you have a long half-life drug, its kinetics may not be the same across the time curve. Data show that urinary excretions differ from day to night. A paper I presented in 1962 in Dallas had a graph which showed (not my data) that when hydropenic people – those who lack water – go from ambulatory to bedridden, the urinary pH and ammonia rise. We are about to check this out in normal people. The point is, that there is a difference between ambulatory and bedridden people but the difference is not known quantitatively. In case of a drug whose pK is near the urinary pH, a half pH unit change in urine can make a fantastic difference in back diffusion of certain drugs.

Question (audience): I have detected a difference of opinion in the panel today on whether you can use urine data as opposed to blood data. Dr. *Wagner*, you have established blood-urine correlations and did a major part of your work with urine data, would you comment?

Response (Dr. Wagner): During 7 years of study, whenever I calculated bioavailability from the area under blood level curve – corrected or uncorrected – or from the total amount excreted in urine, the answers were usually within 3 % of each other. This was done measuring unchanged drug and under very carefully controlled conditions of diet, etc.

Comment (Dr. Levy): If you have a drug whose renal clearance is highly pH dependent and which is subject to several parallel and competing pathways, you must be very careful with urinary studies. It depends on the type of assay – specific or nonspecific – whether you can account for all of the drug in one form or another in the urine. The problem that one faces is to find the kind of facility that will give you the properly timed and frequent enough blood or plasma samples to get a good area under the curve. Sometimes you can get better cooperation and tighter protocols with urinary execution studies. I must emphasize that one cannot generalize – it depends on the drug and the conditions of trial.

Comment (Dr. Riegelman): With regard to the assay of total radioactivity in urine and blood studies, I wish to emphasize the hazards and lack of sensitivity. With such methods one sees all metabolites as well as the intact drug. Rarely do metabolite and intact drugs have the same distribution and elimination characteristics as the drug itself. One obtains only a rough evaluation of the drug absorbed by such methodology.

Question (audience): I detect a slight difference of opinion between panel members on the question of whether to use healthy volunteers or clinical patients in bioavailability studies. I believe we should use healthy volunteers to keep variables at a minimum. I would like to hear more about this.

Response (Dr. Levy): There is not much disagreement. The point is that sometimes one encounters problems in patients that are not encountered in normal subjects. We should address ourselves to the actual situation. The regular monitoring of blood in patients is good medical practice and here is an opportunity to retest periodically those drugs already in the market and to test the generic equivalence of those entering it. To be sure you do not have a totally unabsorbed compound, an initial trial of the new product on a small number of healthy subjects should be conducted. Then, to document bioavailability, go to a patient population on determined steady states. Your assay must be rapid enough so that you know when the plateau level is moving even slightly and you can discontinue and return to the readily-available drug.

Question (Dr. Azarnoff): Is it not true that you would pick up the same information on a single-dose study?

Response (Dr. Levy): Not necessarily. Some products are absorbed over a long period of time and will show a long tailing in plasma concentration. This may not be recognized because drug concentration is lower than detectable. If the same drug is given repeatedly one may not get any difference between two products. I am just advocating maximum utilization of the facilities that we have.

Comment (Dr. Azarnoff): Yes, I agree but I am speaking specifically of digoxin.

Comment (Dr. Wagner): I must disagree with Dr. *Levy.* I had a study where 0.1 mg digitoxin was administered and plasma level was studied for 15 days. Now no drug is absorbed beyond 15 days – most are absorbed within 48 hours. I do not believe that a multiple dose curve gives you that much more information. Most studies I performed in industry were multiple-dose studies. In this way you do not have to know anything about pharmacokinetics. The area you measure within one dosage internal is independent and it is not necessary to extrapolate to infinity. Extrapolation can be wrong, when you do not have first-order kinetics. To get around this problem, do a multiple dose study, but not on sick patients because you cannot control them well enough. For example, an average sick patient receives 14 drugs in 14 days.

Question (audience): In your digoxin slide you showed different capabilities of compounds based on the same weight. Are you prepared in the case of levels to recommend that there be a whole series of doses of the accepted reference product which delivers say, $66^2/_3$ or 77 % of the new product? Because we have a better new product, must we alter our accepted doses?

Dr. Wagner: I do not understand.

Questioner: According to your slide one must alter accepted doses accordingly.

Response (Dr. Wagner): Let me explain the slide and that may clarify the issue. Preparation A was 0.6 available relative to B. If I have a patient on 0.5 mg per day of A, and I change to B, obviously I have to lower the dose. In US hospitals people are receiving digoxin at 4–10 times normal doses because the tablets are of poor quality.

Comment (Dr. Azarnoff): The purpose of this conference is to establish standards so that this does not happen.

Questioner: He did not answer my question.

Comment (Dr. Azarnoff): Let me try to answer. You are concerned that one product delivers to a patient more drug than another one. This is the purpose of this conference – all formulations of a drug should deliver the same amount of drug. The next question the panel should address itself to is: if a new product delivers more drug than the standard product should it become the new standard?

Comment (Dr. Levy): This is a point I tried to cover in my talk. If a product for some reason is incompletely absorbed, the variation from subject to subject and within subjects from day to day is tremendous. Do all you can to obtain essentially complete bioavailability by suitable formulation; as soon as you know that there is an incomplete bioavailability problem, act accordingly. Spironolactone is an example where the company acted responsibly and reformulated their product so as to decrease dosage. Some brands are more extensively absorbed than the innovator's product. Now it would be folly to misformulate, to bring new products to the lower quality of the innovator's in this case. We should have a common denominator of quality with regard to bioavailability.

Comment (Dr. Azarnoff): Do I understand correctly that there may be a product with greater bioavailability for patients with a certain disease as compared to normal man?

Comment (Dr. Levy): I am glad you brought this up. In times of insecurity there is the tendency to equalize everything so we do not have to use discriminating judgment. In principle, I do not care for this kind of approach. This notion of equality is regressive, it impedes the development of excellence in drug products. Although I do not see much of this happening, I visualize the possibility that different kinds of dosage forms of a given drug may be suited to different kinds of patients.

Comment (Dr. Riegelman): I wish to rephrase Dr. *Azarnoff*'s question and expand it beyond the question of bioavailability. The rate and extent of absorption will affect the way that a drug acts and we should probably modify the dosage forms to suit particular disease states.

Comment (Dr. Wagner): You study five dosage forms of a product and plot *in vivo* data in man versus an *in vitro* parameter such as dissolution time. Find out the duration of the plateau level since this is unique for each drug and dosage form. Then in a certain range you can make lot to lot changes with no effect on bioavailability. Under such circumstances you can apply *in vitro* specifications to bioavailability based on good science.

Question (audience): Dr. *Fales,* what is the capacity of the amberlite resin you mentioned and would it be possible to separate enough urinary metabolites for examination by thin layer chromatography followed by NMR?

Response (Dr. Fales): Yes, capacity is reasonably high. It is used for routine drug analyses – heroin in urine. One can obtain mg quantities.

Comment (Dr. Azarnoff): Would you care to comment on ion-pair extraction as a means of purifying drugs.

Comment (Dr. Fales): No, I do not have any personal experience in that area.

Question (audience): Would there be any bearing on bioavailability by changing from dosage by weight, to dosage by surface area?

Response (Dr. Wagner): Absolutely not. I studied this some time ago. If you plot surface area versus body weight, the two are very highly correlated, 0.95 or better, in a range of adult body weight, 120–180 lbs. If you compare children to man, or mice or rats to man, it may be better to relate dosage to surface area.

Question (audience): We know there are individual differences between people – metabolism, diet, environment, blood levels, etc. Have effects from these been observed with drugs studied?

Response (Dr. Levy): It is important to remember that bioavailability is affected by the dosage form, and that elimination kinetics and distribution are not ordinarily dosage-form effects. But one should be knowledgeable about these. If a drug is rapidly and completely absorbed, it is not very sensitive to these factors.

Comment (Dr. Barr): I would like to mention factors which influence intestinal metabolism. Salicylic acid inhibits salicylamide metabolism by two different routes – competitive, glucuronide formation and non-competitive, sulfate formation. It is quite possible that other drugs in combination with salicylamide and aspirin may influence intestinal metabolism of each other.

Question (audience): There is some confusion between comparative bioavailability and comparative pharmacokinetics. It seems to me that the only logical way to study bioavailability of two products is in a crossover study using normal subjects. Then you can set parameters when designing a new formulation.

Response (Dr. Wagner): Unless you study all physiologic factors and drug interactions that may affect the fate of a drug you cannot design good bioavailability studies.

Comment (Dr. Riegelman): To do some of these studies one must cross the realm of clinical pharmacokinetics.

Comment (Dr. Barr): It is a matter of semantics. The problem is to identify those formulation factors which alter pharmacological effects or interactions with any physiologic event that can alter pharmacological effect. To design a study you must first find a sensitive method to evaluate two or three formulations in healthy people. This will not necessarily be clinically significant.

Comment (Dr. Levy): If I understand the question correctly – here we are trying to evaluate two or three formulations – why not evaluate in healthy subjects in a crossover experiment and get the answer? Normal subjects on empty stomachs do give reproducible results. However, the point is not to get the cleanest test conditions but the most predictable and representative conditions to give you the kind of answers you need. Quite often two products will not show differences under ideal conditions but they will under clinical conditions.

Question (audience): I would like some clarification on studying blood levels of a drug over several half-lives. This may take weeks.

Response (Dr. Wagner): For drugs with half-lives up to 24 h it is reasonable to do single-dose studies; when half-life is greater, multiple-dose studies are more reasonable.

Question (audience): I was quite surprised to hear Dr. *Levy* say that he advocates different kinds of drugs, some well absorbed, some not so well absorbed, etc.

Response (Dr. Levy): I think you have misunderstood me. At no time have I advocated the marketing of drugs that are incompletely absorbed as a result of purposeful formulation. I mentioned the design of special dosage forms that would meet the needs of special patients such as elderly persons or persons with a malabsorption problem.

Comment (Dr. Weiner): I think there is some confusion regarding two facets of bioavailability – completeness of absorption and speed of absorption. The latter can vary with the patient. But nobody wants an incompletely absorbed drug since there is no control over dose. However, the speed of absorption can be varied to meet the need of the patient; here is the area for innovation.

Comment (Dr. Riegelman): The comment is well taken. We want some drugs to be absorbed relatively slowly so they do not peak too high. Also some drugs that are absorbed too fast do not render sufficient therapeutic effect.

Comment (Dr. Wagner): Just because two products are 100 % bioavailable does not mean that they have equal efficacy. Take, for example, sodium tolbutamide and tolbutamide, each 1 g per tablet. Using the acid form, one obtains a large area under the blood sugar curve; using the sodium salt, the area is only half as much.

Question (audience): I am concerned about drugs that are not completely absorbed, such as the quarternary ammonium compounds mentioned by Dr. *Levy.* These can be formulated to change the degree of absorption by several orders of magnitude by the addition of additives. How many compounds are really candidates of this sort?

Response (Dr. Levy): I am also concerned about the variability. Drugs that are potent and variably absorbed are obviously poor candidates for oral administration for reasons of safety and efficacy. We are focusing on a number of compounds that are poorly absorbed from solution, but present no dissolution-rate problem, by using two approaches – increasing the viscosity and use of anticholinergic agents to increase absorption. We find it is not possible; variability increases as the absorption rate is increased. In the case of the acid-sensitive penicillins, we wish to retain the drug in the solid state in the stomach and have it rapidly dissolve in the intestines. One must use risk/benefit ratio judgment, but compounds that have an unfavorable therapeutic ratio are poor candidates for oral administration if absorbed variably.

Pharmacology 8: 153–198 (1972)

Panel Discussion on Case Histories in Bioavailability of Drugs

Moderator: *J.T. Doluisio,* Lexington, Ky. (USA)
Participants: *L.J. Leeson,* Summit, N.J. (USA); *A.J. Glazko,* Ann Arbor, Mich. (USA); *J.D. Conklin,* Norwich, N.Y. (USA); *R.A. O'Reilly,* San Jose, Calif. (USA); *D. Cook,* Ottawa, Ont. (Canada)

Introductory Remarks of the Moderator

J.T. Doluisio
Department of Pharmacology, University of Kentucky, Lexington, Ky.

There are those who seem to feel that drug products from different manufacturers which contain the same amount of pure active ingredient will perform identically. This is wrong. For example, I could prepare one tablet of drug using the purest milk sugar in the formulation and a second tablet using powdered cement. Both could contain the correct amount of pure drug and be termed generic equivalents. I am certain you would not want anyone to take the tablet containing the cement.

You might say this is an absurd example, and it is, but it certainly does point to the fact that label or assay is often inadequate. Certainly no reputable manufacturer would use cement in a product but indeed he does make many decisions on how he will manufacture a drug product and in some cases the wrong decision would be equivalent to adding cement to the formulation. A drug product not only consists of the drug itself but it also consists of fillers, binding agents, lubricants, etc., all of which can affect the performance of the drug product. For example, lubricants are used to make powder free-flowing during the manufacturing process. The more lubricant, the easier the product is to mass-produce. However, too much lubricant may raincoat the powder and prevent the drug from being dissolved in the gastrointestinal tract and absorbed into the body. Consequently, even though the labeled amount of pure drug is present in the dosage form the product may have a poor performance, and in effect may be subpotent. It is abundantly clear that there is much potential to alter drug absorption characteristics during the manufacture of a dosage form.

There are often official standards regulating the manufacture of drug products. Unfortunately, at present these standards are only adequate with respect to insuring chemical equivalence. They emphasize such things as purity of the drug, stability in the dosage form, assay versus labeled potency, tablet to tablet or unit to unit variation, etc.

At present, there are no enforced standards which will insure bioavailability. One thus encounters products on the market which indeed fulfill all requirements for chemical equivalence but which are potentially inefficient with respect to their therapeutic effect in the body. Only the ultimate development of proper standards will insure that drug products are equivalent in all respects. This is why we are here.

Certains drugs, and certain dosage forms, are more likely to cause formulation problems than others. Formulating a drug product is more difficult when it contains only minute quantities of drug. In this case the mixing of tablet ingredients for example must be very thorough to insure that the drug is uniformly distributed throughout the powder mass prior to compression of the tablet. In the spring of 1970, many formulations of digoxin were withdrawn from the market for containing both sub- and superpotent tablets in the same bottle. This was a result of inefficient mixing during the manufacturing process.

Another drug factor to consider is the solubility of the chemical form of the drug. Drugs of low aqueous solubility would have the greatest potential for having variations in apparent absorption.

It is obvious that dosage forms in which the drug is farthest from aqueous solution have the greatest potential for variation in biologic availability. Consequently, we may expect that the risk of differences in bioavailability varies to some degree with the type of dosage form involved. A dosage form that has the drug in solution such as an elixir would have a relatively low potential for differences in biologic availability. Dosage forms that have the drug in a subdivided solid state, such as a suspension or a capsule or a chewable tablet, would probably have an intermediate potential. And a dosage form that has the drug in a compacted state, such as a compressed tablet, or in even more complicated systems such as sustained-release dosage forms or enteric-coated dosage forms, would have probably the highest potential for biologic inequivalency.

Today's panel will discuss some 'case histories' in bioavailability of certain drugs when formulated in dosage forms.

We look forward to a stimulating session – one in which we hope you will actively participate. Our panel will discuss the four drugs listed in the program. Members of the audience may participate by responding to or questioning the panel – or they may wish to present data from their own studies.

We have asked our panel speakers to limit their remarks to 10 min – no panel speaker will be allowed more than 15 min.

Author's address: Prof. *James T. Doluisio,* Chairman, Department of Pharmacology, University of Kentucky, Washington and Gladstone Streets, *Lexington, KY 40506* (USA)

Phenylbutazone

L.J. Leeson
Department of Pharmacy Research, Ciba-Geigy, Summit, N.J.

In the past 10–15 years, with the greater awareness of bioavailability, phenylbutazone has been one of the drugs receiving considerable attention in this regard. The *in vivo/in vitro* studies by *Searl and Pernarowski* (1), as well as those by *Van Petten et al.* (2) are examples of such work. In addition, as early as 1953 (3) some experimenters compared the availability of various phenylbutazone dosage forms. Today, I would like to discuss with you our experience in developing an improved phenylbutazone tablet.

The poor solubility and wettability characteristics of phenylbutazone make it a drug with which one might expect to encounter availability problems. Therefore, a few years ago,

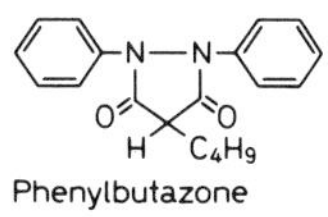

a

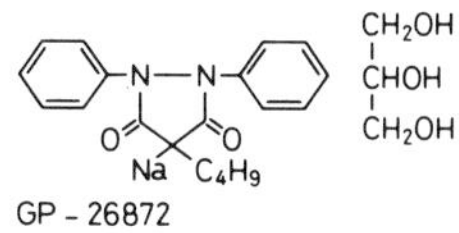

b

Fig. 1a and 1b: Phenylbutazone and Na-salt of phenylbutazone monoglyceride (GP-26872).

when a salt of phenylbutazone with high solubility became available to us, it appeared to offer the potential for developing a better dosage form of phenylbutazone. This compound (GP-26872), which is the sodium salt of phenylbutazone, is crystallized as the monoglyceride (fig. 1).

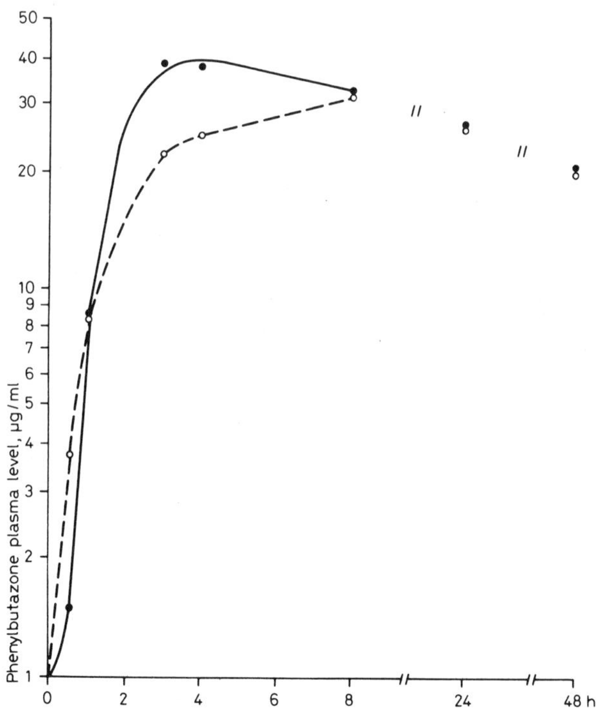

Fig. 2. ○ = GP-26872; ● = Phenylbutazone.

Table I.

Parameter	Butazolidin	GP-26872
$\frac{k_{ab}\,Df}{(k_{ab}-K)\,V_p}$ (γ/ml)	35.4	34.3
t_l, h	0.50	0.32
K, h^{-1}	0.0112	0.0112
k_{ab}, h^{-1}	0.705	0.390
Time for total absorption, h	3.0	5.3

In an initial crossover study involving 20 patients, phenylbutazone and GP-26872 capsule formulations were compared. The plasma level curves obtained in this study are shown in figure 2. It may be seen that although during the first half hour the plasma levels appear to be better for the soluble GP-26872, shortly after this the curves cross over, resulting in the phenylbutazone reaching a higher level earlier. The two capsules were found to be equally available by an area under the curve comparison. In addition, a simple pharmacokinetic analysis of this data was performed assuming a one-compartment open model with first-order absorption. The equation employed is seen in the following formula:

$$C_p = \frac{k_{ab}\cdot f\cdot D}{(k_{ab}-K)\,V_p}\left[e^{-K(t-t_l)}-e^{-k_{ab}(t-t_l)}\right],$$

where C_p = plasma concentration; k_{ab} = pseudo: first-order absorption, rate constant K = elimination rate constant; t = time; t_l = lag time; D = administered dose; f = fraction absorbed; V_p = volume of distribution.

The terminology defined in this formula is typical of that which is routinely employed in this type of study. The term t_l is a lag time term we have introduced to account for the initial delay in onset at plasma levels. These parameters were evaluated employing the method of *Wagner and Nelson* and are shown in table I. The pertinent data of interest to us are the absorption rate constants. These were unexpectedly opposite in magnitude from what had been predicted, based on the solubility of the respective forms of phenylbutazone. That is, the higly soluble GP-26872, demonstrated an apparent first-order rate constant, almost half of that obtained with the less soluble phenylbutazone free acid. The time required for the total drug to be absorbed is also in qualitative agreement with this.

In an effort to understand these somewhat unexpected results, we performed *in vitro* dissolution determinations on the capsules, employing the USP XVIII (rotating basket) apparatus. The results of this study (fig. 3) indicate that the dissolution curves bear a remarkable similarity to the plasma level absorption curves in that initially the GP-26872 capsule demonstrated the more rapid dissolution rate, but after a short time the rate decreased resulting in a longer time for total drug to be released. An observation of the physical behavior of the dissoluting GP-26872 capsule indicated a poorly dispersing formulation, which, in turn, resulted in a poor release rate for the active ingredient. Employing t_{90}, the time for 90 % of the drug to be released during *in vitro* dissolution, as a measure of dissolution rate, there is an interesting correlation between *in vivo* absorption rate constant and *in vitro* dissolution rate. This is shown in table II. While the excellent correspondence of the ratios obtained for either the absorption rate constants, or the times for total drug absorption, and the *in vitro* dissolution rates are somewhat fortuitous, we felt these results indicated that the absorption problem with this soluble form of drug was related to its release from the dosage form. Dissolution measurements of pure GP-26872 and phenylbutazone demonstrated that our formulations had a large affect on the release of the active ingredient.

Table II.

System	k_{ab}, h^{-1}	t_{ab}, h	t_{90}, min	$\frac{k_{ab}(B)}{k_{ab}(G)}$	$\frac{t_{ab}(G)}{t_{ab}(B)}$	$\frac{t_{90}(G)}{t_{90}(B)}$
Butazolidin (B)	0.705	3.0	58	1.8	1.8	1.8
GP-26872 (G)	0.390	5.3	106			

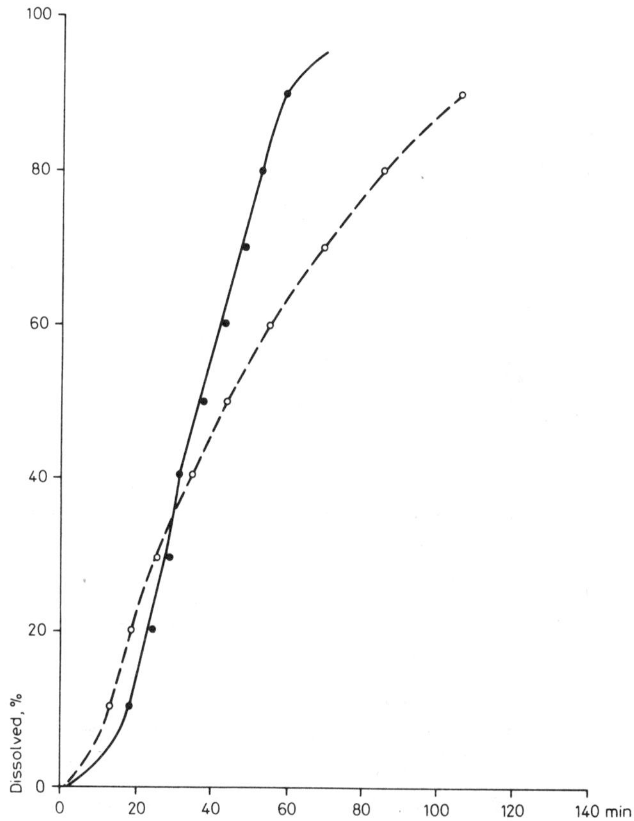

Fig. 3. ○ = GP-26872; ● = Phenylbutazone.

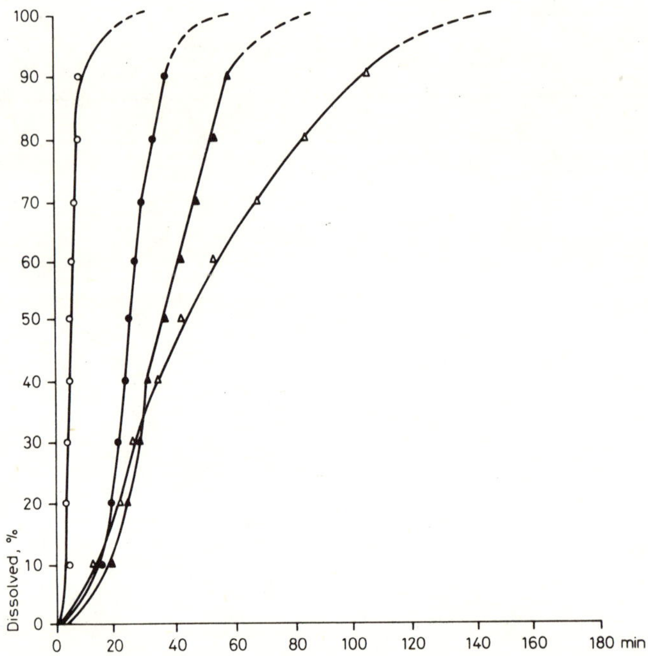

Fig. 4. ○ = GP-26872 AI; ● = Butazolidin AI; △ = GP-26872 formulated; ▲ = Butazolidin formulated.

This is shown in figure 4 along with the original dissolution data for the formulated capsules and indicates that the GP-26872 was especially influenced in a negative way by the formulation.

If, as we previously concluded, the dissolution rate was the controlling absorption of these compounds, then the pure GP-26872 active ingredient should demonstrate an absorption rate superior to pure phenylbutazone. In a crossover study involving 13 patients and employing only active ingredients in capsules, the following plasma level curves were obtained (fig. 5). It is apparent that in addition to demonstrating far more rapid absorption than the pure phenylbutazone, the GP-26872 showed measurable blood levels at the end of 15 min, something that had never before been encountered with phenylbutazone. Furthermore, the patient-to-patient variation at any point was statistically significantly lower for the soluble salt of phenylbutazone than it was for the less soluble free acid. However, as with the previous study, the area under the curve values indicated essentially equal availability from both capsules.

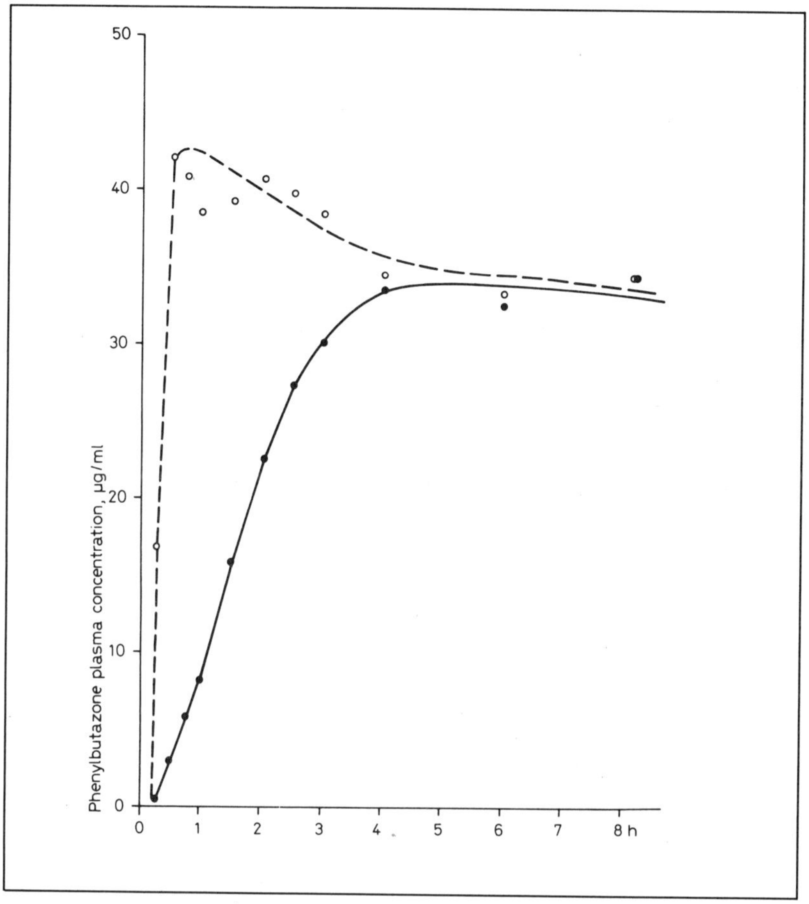

Fig. 5. ○ = GP-26872; ● = Phenylbutazone.

Our next problem was related to developing a workable GP-26872 capsule formulation which demonstrated rapid *in vitro* dissolution. The *in vitro* dissolution behavior of the product which we developed is shown in figure 6. We felt that its dissolution rate was sufficiently similar to pure GP-26872 to mimic its *in vivo* behavior. For comparative purposes, I have included in figure 6 the dissolution curve for the commercial Butazolidin tablet being sold at that time. In a crossover study involving 20 patients, serum levels were determined for this new formulation in comparison to that for the commercial Butazolidin sugar-coated tablet (fig. 7). As in the previous study with active ingredients, measurable plasma levels were obtained as early as 15 min, and peak levels within $^1/_2-1$ h. In addition, the patient-to-patient variation at each point was statistically significantly smaller than that of the commercial product.

Concomitantly with the above studies, we had been considering ways to improve the absorption rate of phenylbutazone itself by introducing formulation modifications which

6

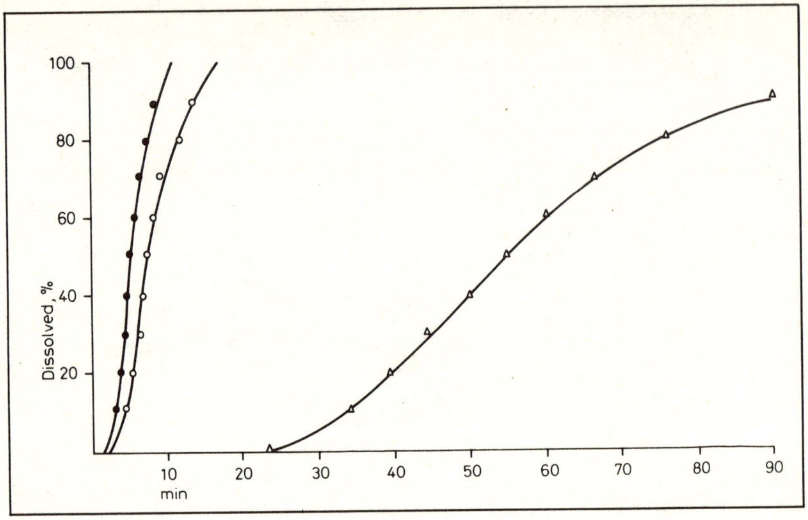

7

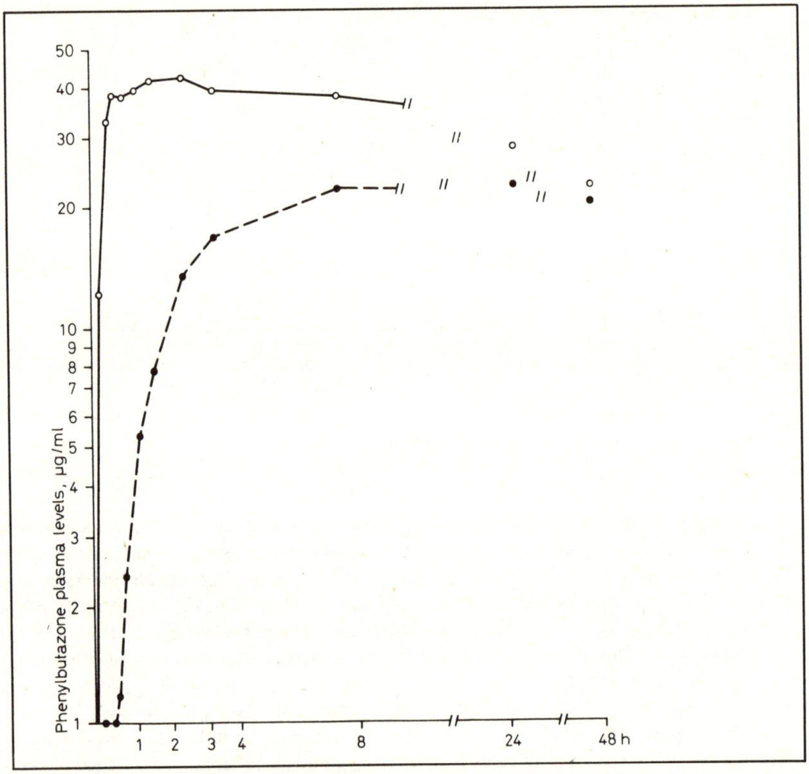

Fig. 6. ● = GP-26872 active ingredient; ○ = GP-26872 capsule formulation; Δ = Phenylbutazone tablets.

Fig. 7. ○ = Na-PB; ● = PB commercial.

8

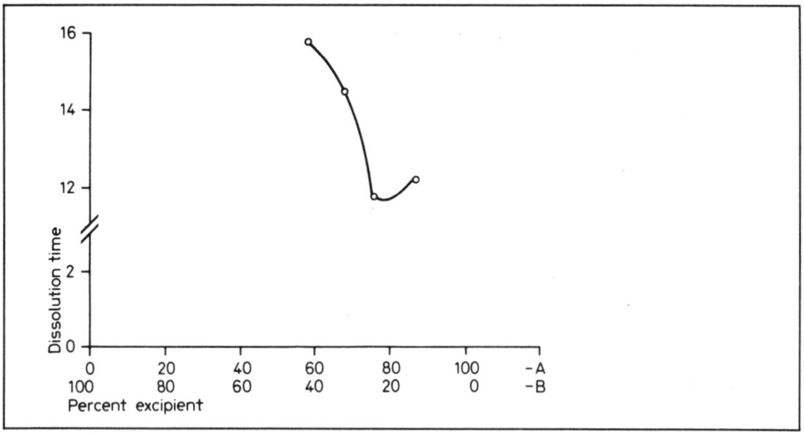

9

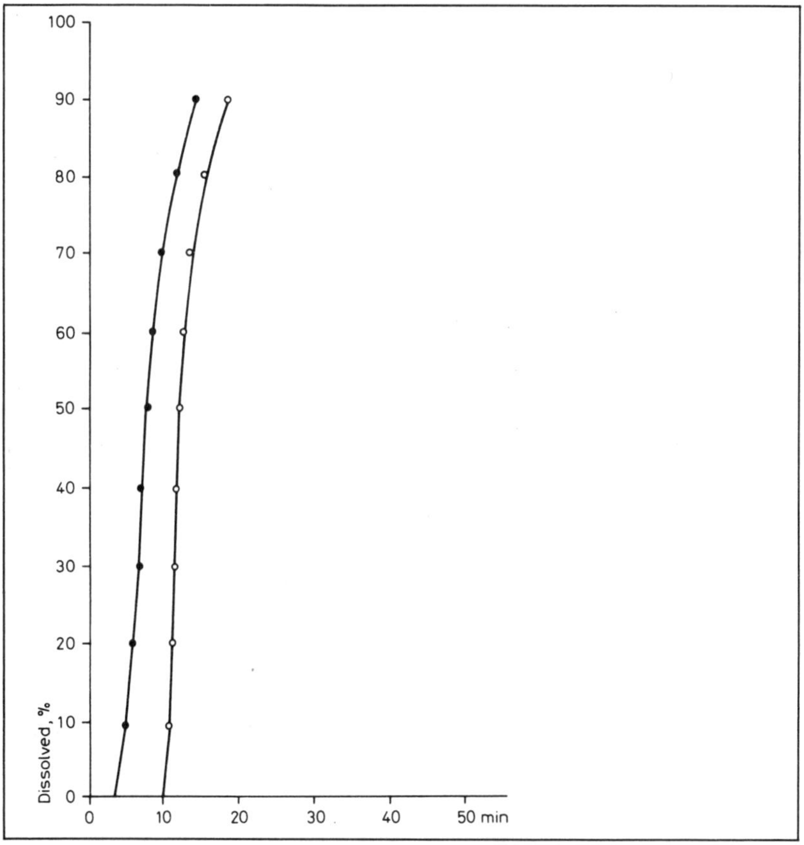

Fig. 8. Dissolution rate of GP-26872 containing various proportions of two excipients.

Fig. 9. ● = GP-26872 formulation; ○ = Butazolidin film tablets.

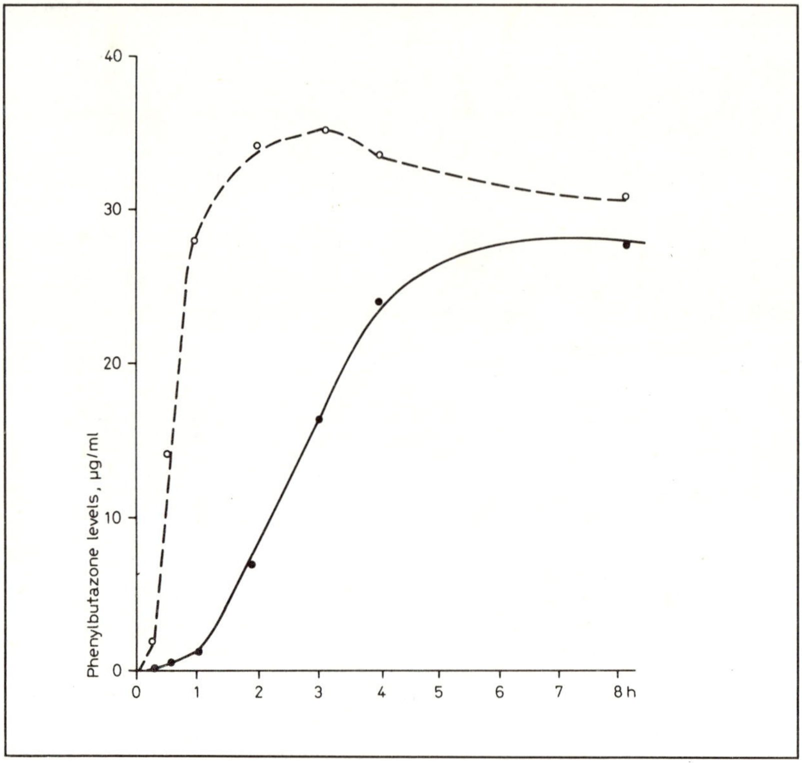

Fig. 10. ○ = Film-coated tablet; ● = Sugar-coated tablet.

would yield more rapid *in vitro* dissolution. It had been determined that two particular formulation ingredients which were used as excipients appeared to aid in the dissolution of this product when certain manufacturing techniques were employed. A series of tablet formulations were prepared containing various amounts of these two ingredients, and the resulting tablets were compared by *in vitro* dissolution rate determinations. The results of this study (fig. 8) indicated that the curve relating dissolution rate with excipient ratio showed a minimum value. This ratio was selected, and film-coated tablets were prepared for evaluation. As can be seen in figure 9, this product's *in vitro* dissolution rate compared favorably with that for the soluble GP-26872 capsule. Blood level values comparing this material to the commercially available tablet at that time are shown in figure 10 and indicate that we had a product which behaved in a manner similar to the more soluble and wettable GP-26872 formulation. There is possibly an additional 15 min time factor associated with blood levels, and peak values occurred anywhere from 1 to 2 h with these film-coated tablets. However, this tablet formulation demonstrated the same statistically significant decrease in variation at each point and was considered to be an excellent product. Thus, we were able to develop a product using the unmodified compound and relying only on formulation variables, without the very real regulatory complexities associated with the marketing of a new salt of a drug.

I hope that our experiences with phenylbutazone demonstrate three important biopharmaceutic concepts. These are certainly not original with us but bear repeating. They are:

(1) A good qualitative *in vitro/in vivo* correlation can be obtained between dosage forms and absorption rate, thus allowing formulations to be developed based on *in vitro* measurements.

(2) As was seen with GP-26872, a poorly designed formulation can destroy the absorption rate of even *highly soluble compounds.* This fact indicates that a capsule formulation, as reported by *Rosen et al.* (5) is not necessarily the ideal form for drug evaluation.

(3) A rapidly absorbed form of even an intrinsically poorly soluble and wettable compound can be obtained by formulation modifications alone.

If I have done little more this morning than to reemphasize these facts, I feel I have accomplished my purpose.

Acknowledgements

The author would like to acknowledge the efforts of his co-workers Mr. *E. Shinal,* Dr. *G. Lukas,* Mrs. *S. Zak* and Dr. *M. Weiner.*

References

1 *Searl, R.O. and Pernarowski, M.:* Canad. med. Ass. J. *96:* 1513 (1967).
2 *Van Petten, G.R. et al.:* J. clin. Pharmacol. *11* (1971).
3 *Burns, J.J. et al.:* J. Pharmacol. exp. Ther. *109:* 346 (1953).
4 *Brodie, B.B. et al.:* Amer. J. Med. *16:* 181 (1954).
5 *Rosen, E. et al.:* Symposium on safer and more effective drugs, Washington, D.C. 1967.

Author's address: Dr. *Lewis J. Leeson,* Assistant Director, Pharmacy Research and Development, Ciba-Geigy, *Summit, NJ 07901* (USA)

Diphenylhydantoin

A.J. Glazko
Chemical Pharmacology Section, Parke, Davis & Company, Ann Arbor, Mich.

Diphenylhydantoin (DPH) presents an intriguing problem in bioavailability because there are so many factors which seem to influence the absorption, distribution and metabolic disposition of this drug. A great deal of new information on the metabolic disposition of DPH has appeared in the last few years, but much remains to be done in this area. Any conclusions we may reach at this time are purely tentative, and hopefully, our minds should remain open for alternative explanations.

You are all aware that different formulations of DPH may show different absorption characteristics. A report before a congressional investigating committee in 1967 indicated that six veteran's hospitals experienced an increase in the number of convulsive seizures when a change was made in the brand of DPH (1), indicating *underdosage* with the new formulation. About the same time, reports from Australia indicated that patients showed signs of *overdosage* when the excipient in the diphenylhydantoin capsules was switched from calcium sulfate to lactose (2, 3). Significant differences in plasma levels were also observed by *Martin et al.* (4) and by *Arnold et al.* (5) following single doses of diphenylhydantoin obtained from different manufacturers. Since this drug is normally given several times a day to epileptic subjects over long periods of time, and as it has a long plasma half-life, and while immediate availability is not an urgent problem, we may be well advised to evaluate such drugs on the basis of repeated dose schedules, rather than to limit our observations to single oral doses.

Figure 1 shows the plasma levels resulting from the peroral administration of different laboratory preparations of diphenylhydantoin to dogs (6). Using equivalent doses, the sodium salt produced higher peak levels at earlier time periods than the acid preparation, which was less soluble in water. The influence of crystal size is clearly indicated by the plasma levels obtained with small and large crystal sizes of DPH.

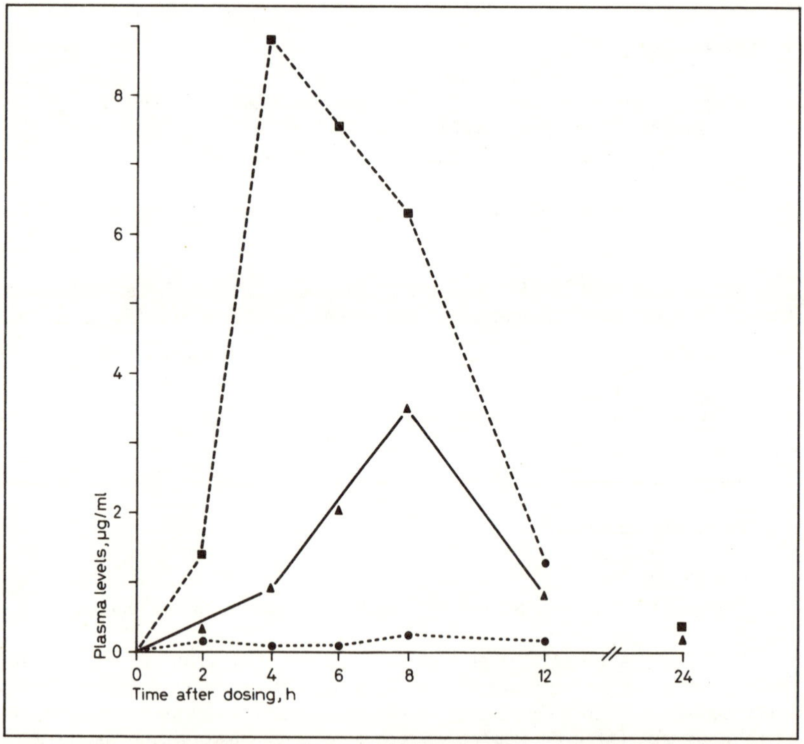

Fig. 1. Dilantin plasma levels, dog, 25 mg/kg p.o. ■ = Dilantin-Na, particle size 5–25 µm; ▲ = dilantin acid, 10–50 µm; ● = dilantin acid, flat plates 0.5 × 3 × 3 mm.

A comparison of plasma levels in 12 normal adult subjects using different formulations of DPH is shown in figure 2. A microcrystalline suspension (Dilantin®, 125 suspension) of the acid form of DPH in 100-mg oral doses produced plasma levels which were nearly identical with those produced by a 100-mg intravenous dose, 4 h after dosing and thereafter. We do not subscribe to the hypothesis that the areas under the two curves must *necessarily* be identical in order to demonstrate completeness of absorption. (a) First, the assay procedure is specific for the parent compound, and does not include metabolites. (b) Secondly, the routes of administration are different. The oral dose passes through the intestinal wall and reaches the liver via the portal circulation; it may be subject to retention and metabolic alteration before entering the systemic circulation. The intravenous dose produces high initial blood levels and may be distributed to other tissues before it reaches the liver. (c) Finally, the slowly rising blood levels following oral dosing, compared with the high initial levels resulting from intravenous administration, may have some effect on the rate of metabolic disposition. This aspect of the problem will be discussed later. In the present study (fig. 2), when the oral doses of the liquid suspension were raised to 200 and 400 mg, the plasma levels appeared to be roughly proportional to dosage. In the final trial, a 400-mg oral dose of Dilantin® sodium kapseals was administered, yielding mean plasma levels only slightly below those observed with the liquid suspension.

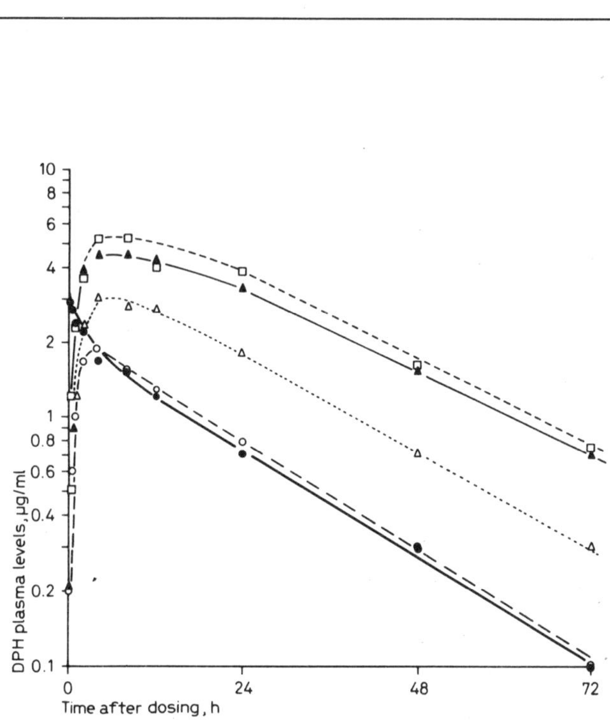

Fig. 2. Dilantin plasma levels, single dose (mean of 12 subjects). ▲ = 400 mg kapseals; □ = 400 mg suspension; △ = 200 mg suspension; ○ = 100 mg suspension; ● = 100 mg i.v.

Table I. ^{14}C-DPH: Balance studies in laboratory animals (i.v. dose = 5 mg/kg; collection period = 72 h)

Species	Dose, %			
	urine	bile	feces	total
Rhesus monkey	88.5	–	6.3	94.8
Bile fistula, monkey	84.4	10.3	0.2	94.9
Beagle dog	80.4	–	20.7	101.1
Bile fistula, dog	54.0	33.6	1.0	88.6

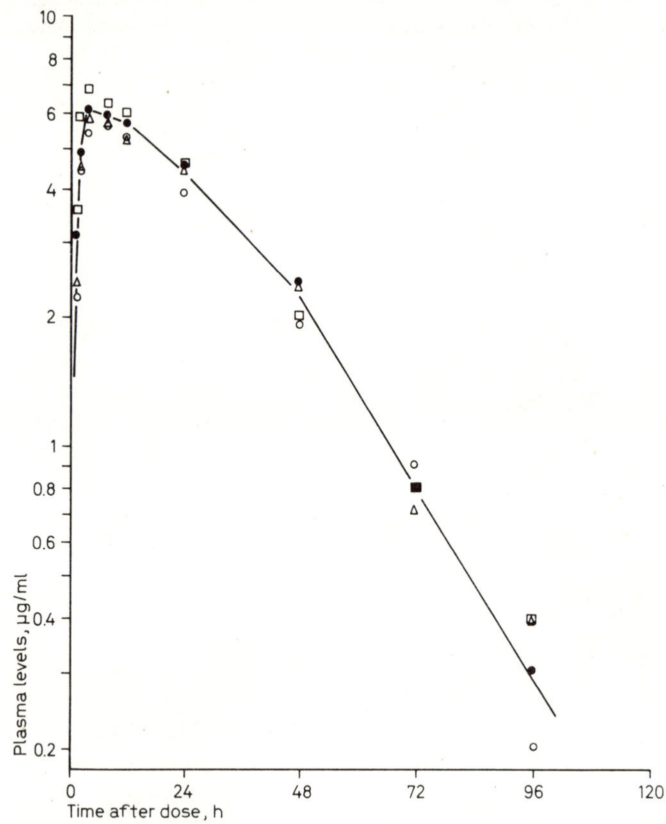

Fig. 3. Mean diphenylhydantoin plasma levels. 4 products, crossover; 0.5 g oral dose (mean of 12 normal subjects). ○ = W; ● = X; △ = Y; □ = Z.

A proper evaluation of absorption from the gastrointestinal tract would require measurement of the residual unabsorbed drug at different time periods after administration. Indirect assays of drug excreted in the feces are complicated by the excretion of metabolites in the bile, and by the possibility of chemical alteration of the drug by bacterial action in the intestinal tract. We carried out balance studies in normal and bile-fistula dogs and monkeys, using 5 mg/kg intravenous doses of ^{14}C-labeled DPH. Urine , bile and feces were collected over a 3-day period, and assayed for total ^{14}C-activity by oxygen flask combustion and liquid scintillation counting. The results are shown in table I. It is evident that biliary excretion is large, with one third of the i.v. dose appearing in dog bile and about 10 % in monkey bile. In the intact animals, about 20 % of the dose appeared in dog feces, and 6 % in monkey feces. Since these values are lower than the biliary excretion data, it seems likely that some of the metabolites excreted in the bile may be reabsorbed. We do not know how much of the drug is excreted in human bile.

In studies which we completed about 3 years ago, DPH capsules from four different manufacturers were administered at weekly intervals to 12 normal adult subjects in single 0.5-gram oral doses, using a Latin square design. The mean plasma levels are shown in figure 3. With preparation Z, 3 subjects showed peak plasma levels 2 h after dosing, but with all 4 preparations, most subjects reached peak plasma levels 4–8 h after dosing, with some taking as long as 12 h. Analysis of variance indicated no significant differences in plasma levels between the treatment groups at the 0.05 level of significance. Note also the apparent change in plasma half-life with time. The plateau out to 12 h is probably due to prolonged absorption of DPH from the intestinal tract; the shorter half-life at the tail end of the curve

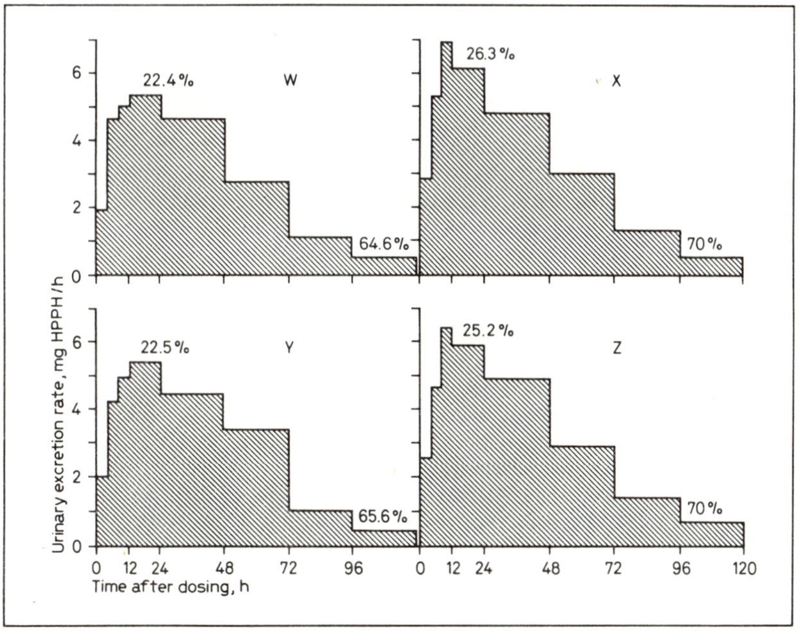

Fig. 4. Mean urinary excretion rate of the four products mentioned in figure 3. Percent figures represent dose recovery.

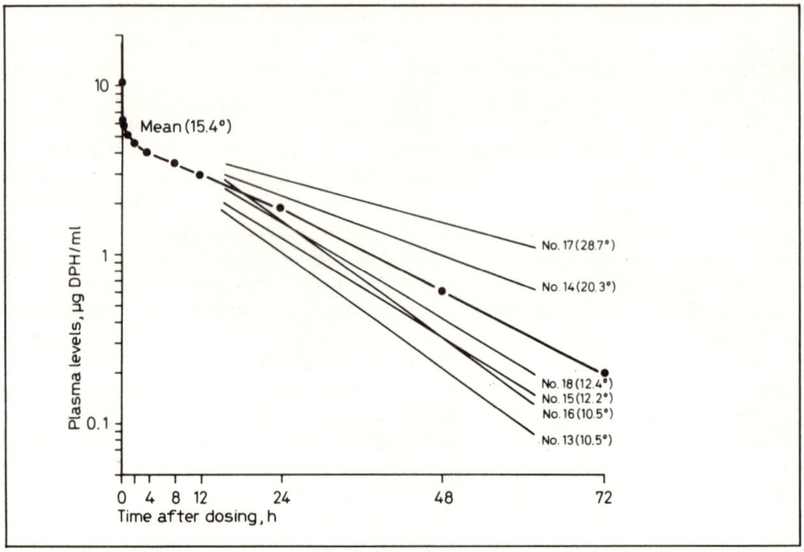

Fig. 5. Plasma levels in normal human subjects following 0.25 g i.v. doses of diphenylhydantoin sodium. Linear regression calculated for the 8- to 72-hour period after dosing; half-lives given in h.

could be due to improper blank corrections. We are convinced that this is not the case. We have seen the same general decrease in half-life with intravenous doses (7), and the same general observations have been made independently by others (8).

Another way to examine the absorption characteristics of a drug is to measure the excretion products. DPH is hydroxylated to form 5-(p-hydroxyphenyl)-5-phenylhydantoin (HPPH), which is conjugated with glucuronic acid and excreted in the urine (9, 10). In the crossover study just described, all urine specimens were assayed for total HPPH by gas-liquid chromatography (11), with the results shown in figure 4. Peak excretion rates occurred in the 8 to 12-hour period after dosing for products X and Z, and in the 12 to 24-hour period for products W and Y. The percent of dose represented by HPPH excretion over a 5-day period was slightly lower for W and Y than for X and Z; however, only two thirds of the dose was accounted for. We do not know the rest of the story on metabolic disposition; it is possible that the excretion of other metabolites which are not detected by this procedure could account for the slight differences noted here. The evidence indicates some differences in absorption rates, but no conclusions can be drawn regarding the true extent of absorption until all of the drug has been accounted for.

Similar data have been obtained following intravenous administration of DPH (7). Plasma levels after 0.25-gram doses are shown in figure 5. The heavy line represents the mean of 6 subjects, and it shows a slight downward inflection. The individual half-lives covered a fairly wide range. In the oral dose series, half-lives for the individual subjects in one series are shown in figure 6, again demonstrating that large variations exist between individuals in their capacity for metabolizing DPH. The urinary excretion of HPPH in the i.v. series is shown in figure 7 with nearly 75 % of the dose being accounted for. This figure ranged from 65 to 81 % of the dose in 5 subjects, and certainly cannot be considered equiva-

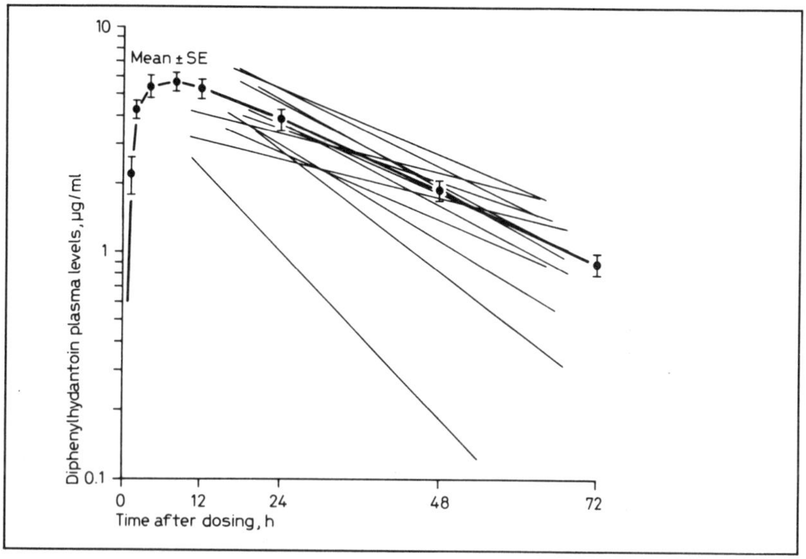

6

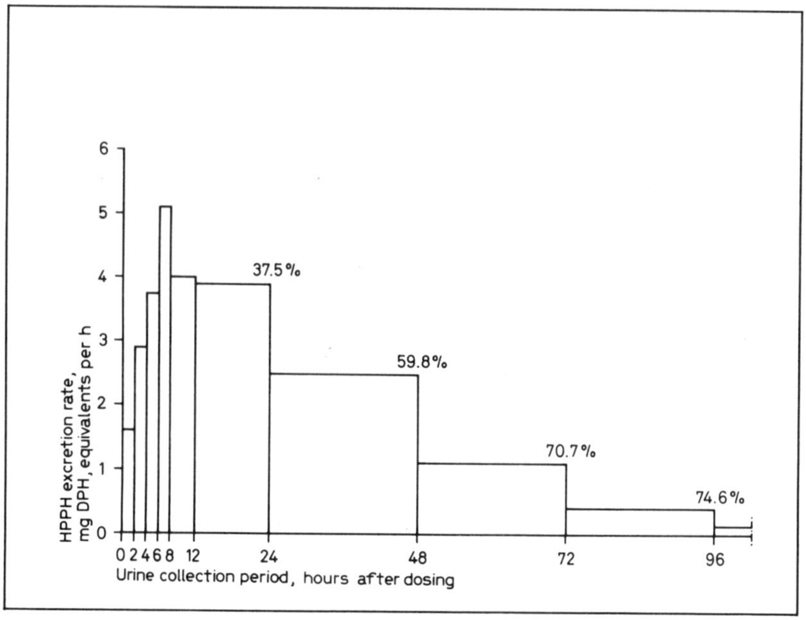

7

Fig. 6. Plasma levels in 12 normal men after single 0.5 g oral doses of dilantin sodium. Linear regression calculated by method of least squares for individual subjects over a 12- to 72-hour period. $t^1/_2$ = 23.5 h; range 9.3–42.2 h.

Fig. 7. Mean HPPH excretion rate in human subjects following 0.25 g i.v. doses of diphenylhydantoin sodium (mean of 5 subjects). Percent figures represent dose recovery.

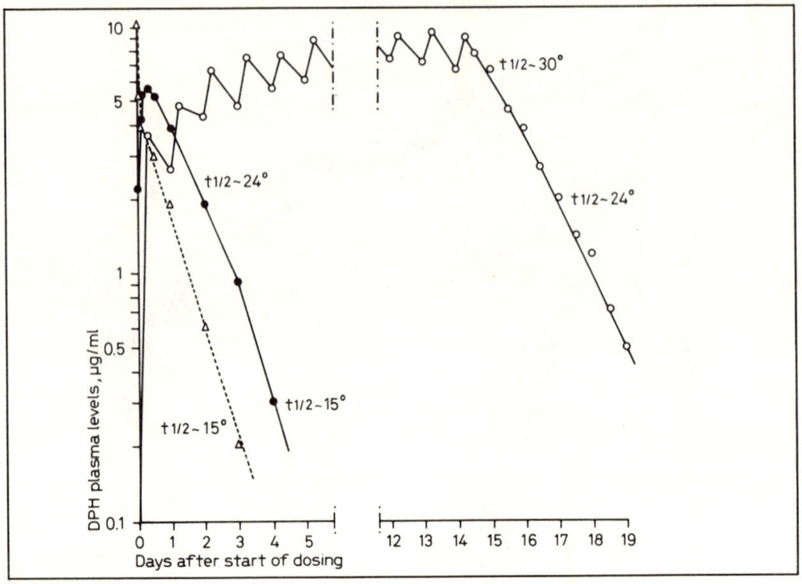

8

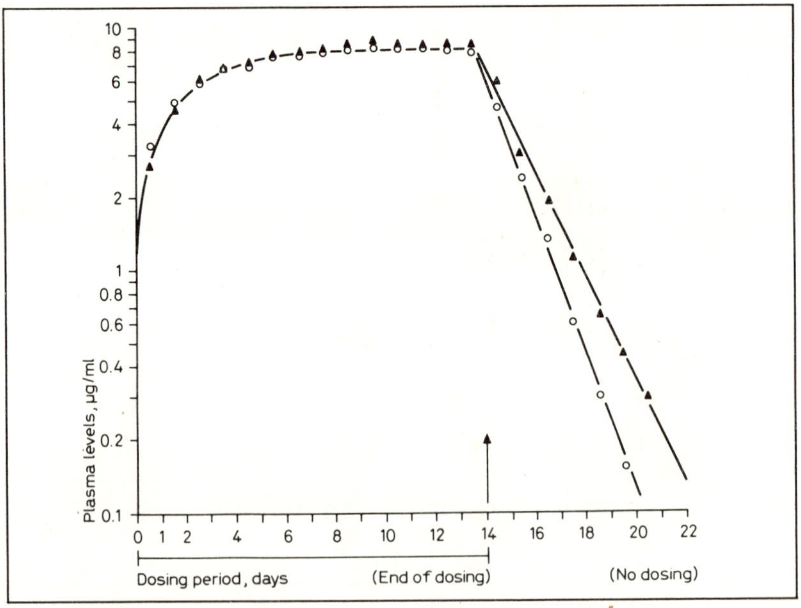

9

Fig. 8. Dilantin plasma levels. △ = 250 mg i.v. dose (mean of 6); ● = 500 mg oral dose (mean of 12); ○ = 300 mg oral dose given once daily for 14 days (mean of 12).

Fig. 9. Dilantin plasma levels, multiple dose (mean of 12 subjects). ▲ = Dilantin kapseals, 100 mg t.i.d.; ○ = dilantin kapseals, 300 mg single dose, once daily.

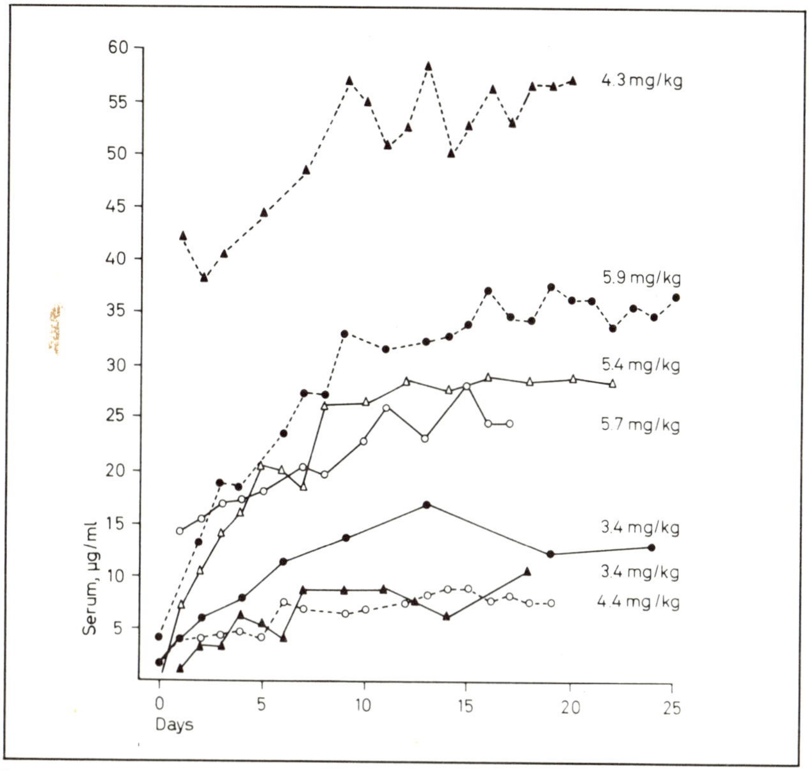

Fig. 10. Serum levels of DPH in 7 patients receiving 300 mg daily doses of DPH. From *Remmer et al.* (13).

lent to an absorption of 100 %. The most significant fact that comes out of this work is that the *urinary excretion of HPPH shows a very marked delay,* with peak excretion rates occurring 6–8 h after the dose has been administered. We will come back to this point later.

In multiple dose trials, 12 subjects were given 300 mg oral doses of DPH once daily for 14 days, with the results shown in figure 8. A period of more than a week was required to reach plateau levels. These were higher than the peak levels following a single 0.5-gram dose. The plasma half-life of DPH also appeared to be greater following termination of dosage, in comparison with the single-dose series. Plasma levels for 300-mg doses given once daily versus the same total daily dose given 100 mg t.i.d. are shown in figure 9. The mean levels (8–9 µg/ml) were about the same for the two dose schedules; individual plateau levels ranged from 3.3 to 17.2 µg/ml. Our clinical trials have demonstrated a good degree of control on once-daily dose schedules (18). However, with the great variation in plasma half-life between subjects, it seems likely that a few patients may require more frequent dosage.

When DPH assay procedures were first developed, we found that some subjects showed consistently high plasma levels of DPH while others were consistently low (12). This is readily evident from plasma level data published recently by *Remmer et al.* (13), shown in

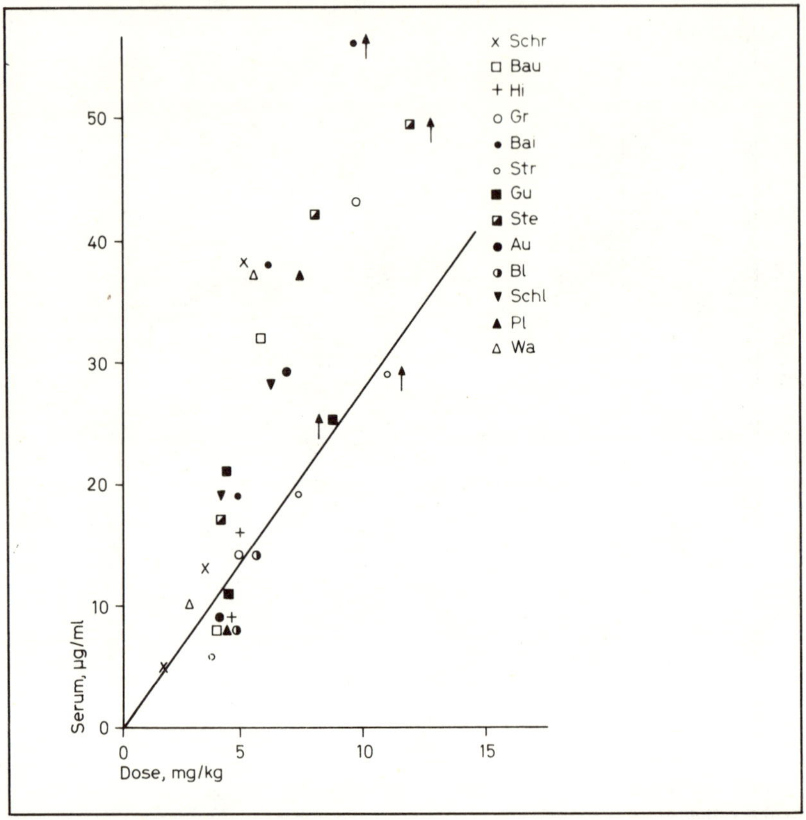

Fig. 11. DPH serum levels in 13 patients maintained initially on 5 mg/kg daily doses of DPH, followed by an increase or decrease in daily dose. Arrows indicate serum levels that were still rising. From *Remmer et al.* (13).

figure 10. At a 300-mg daily dose level, 2 subjects showed plasma levels of 5–10 µg/ml, most were in the range of 10–35 µg/ml, while 1 subject rose to more than 50 µg/ml. *Buchthal et al.* (14) found clinical improvement and normalization of the EEG in the majority of epileptic subjects at DPH plasma levels of 10–20 µg/ml. *Remmer* indicated that changing the daily dose after a constant plasma level had been attained did not always result in a proportionate increase or decrease in plasma levels. As shown in figure 11, only 2 out of

---

Fig. 12. DPH serum levels in 4 patients after termination of dosing (4.3–5 mg/kg daily). From *Remmer et al.* (13).

Fig. 13. The blood half-life of DPH in rats after the i.v. administration of different doses. The half-life is dose dependent. Six rats were studied at each dose and each point represents the mean (± SE) of the levels of DPH in the blood at each time. ○ = 40 mg/kg; △ = 25 mg/kg; □ = 10 mg/kg. From *Gerber et al.* (8).

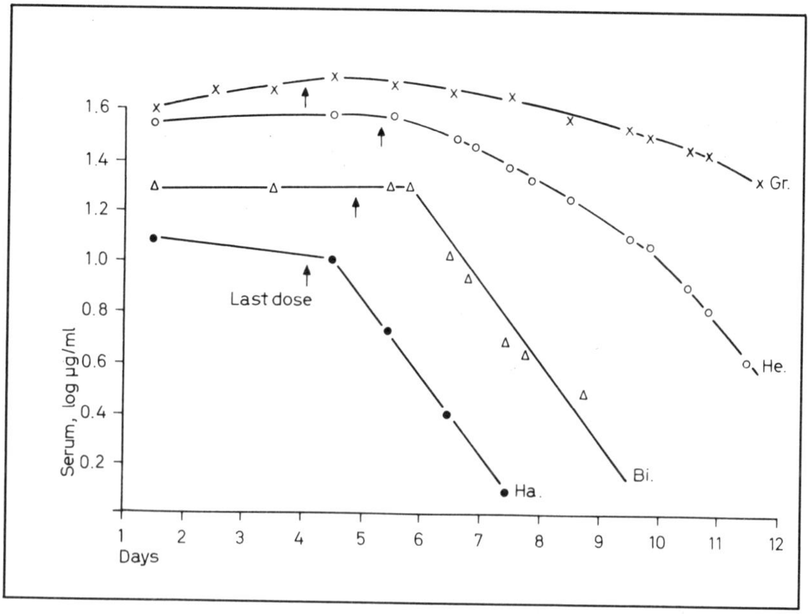
1.6
1.4
1.2
1.0
0.8
0.6
0.4
0.2
Serum, log µg/ml
Last dose
x Gr.
He.
Bi.
Ha.
1 2 3 4 5 6 7 8 9 10 11 12
Days

12

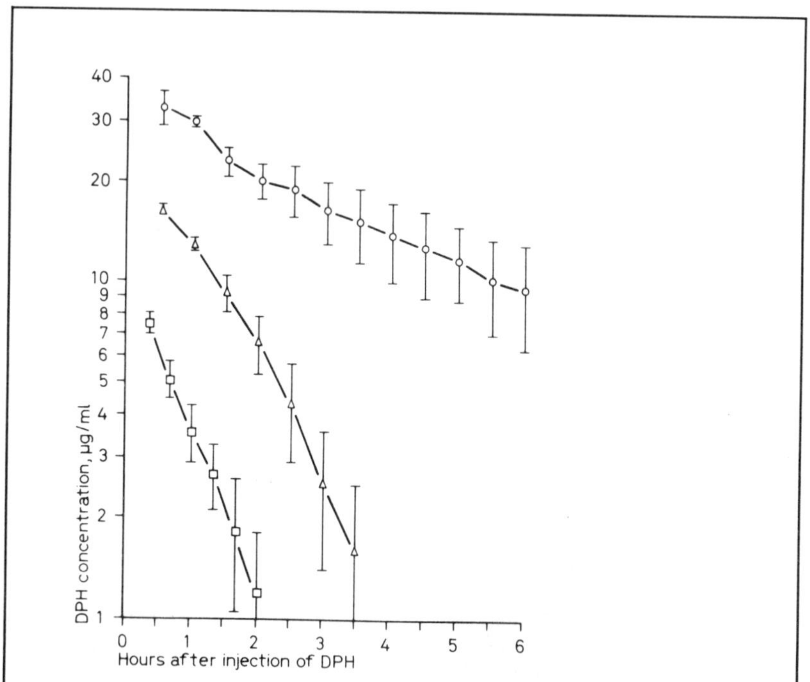
40
30
20
10
9
8
7
6
5
4
3
2
1
DPH concentration, µg/ml
0 1 2 3 4 5 6
Hours after injection of DPH

13

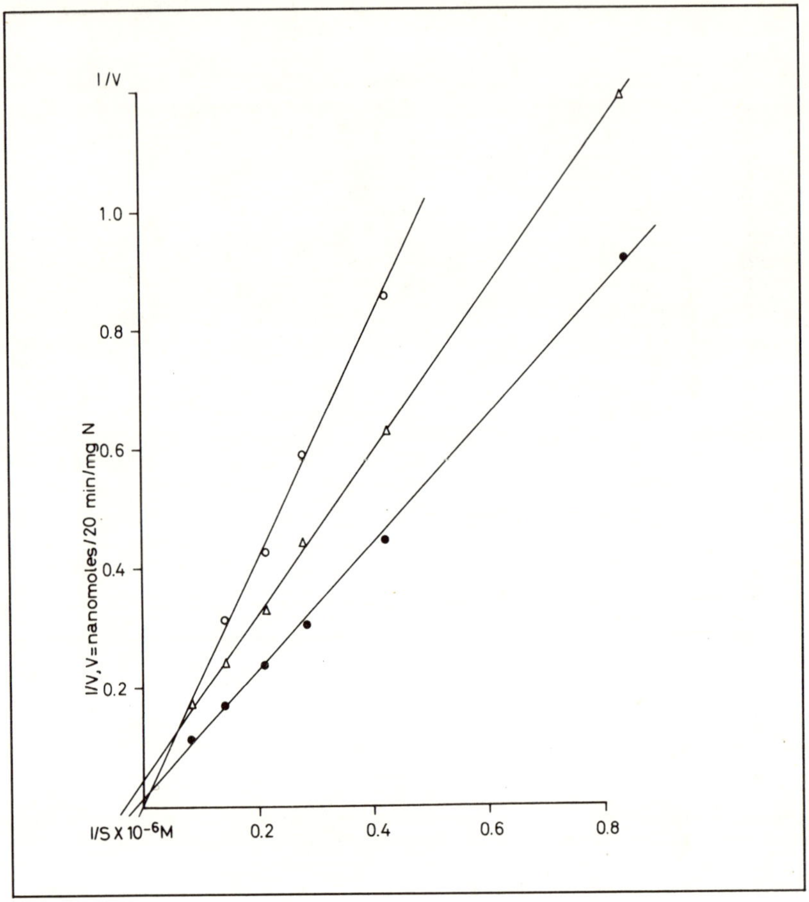

Fig. 14. Inhibition of DPH hydroxylation by synthetic p-HPPH. DPH-^{14}C concentration range 1.2–15 $\times$ 10^{-6}M. HPPH concentration: ○ = 6 $\times$ 10^{-5}M; △ = 3 $\times$ 10^{-5}M; ● = no HPPH added.

13 patients showed changes in plasma levels which were directly proportional to dosage; most subjects showed much higher levels than expected on the basis of dosage. When dosage was terminated, the plasma level drop was nearly exponential only when the levels did not exceed 20–25 μg/ml; above that level, the rate of elimination of DPH appeared to be constant. *Remmer*'s observations are shown in figure 12. The tailing effects were similar to our observations which were made at much lower plasma levels. *Dayton et al.* (15) first reported a dose dependency of plasma DPH levels in dogs. *Arnold and Gerber* (16) and *Gerber and Arnold* (17) also reported that the plasma half-life of DPH in mice and in human subjects was dose dependent. Recent data obtained in the rat are shown in figure 13 (8) with apparent DPH half-lives of 2.5, 1.2 and 0.6 h for i.v. doses of 40.25 and 10 mg/kg, respectively.

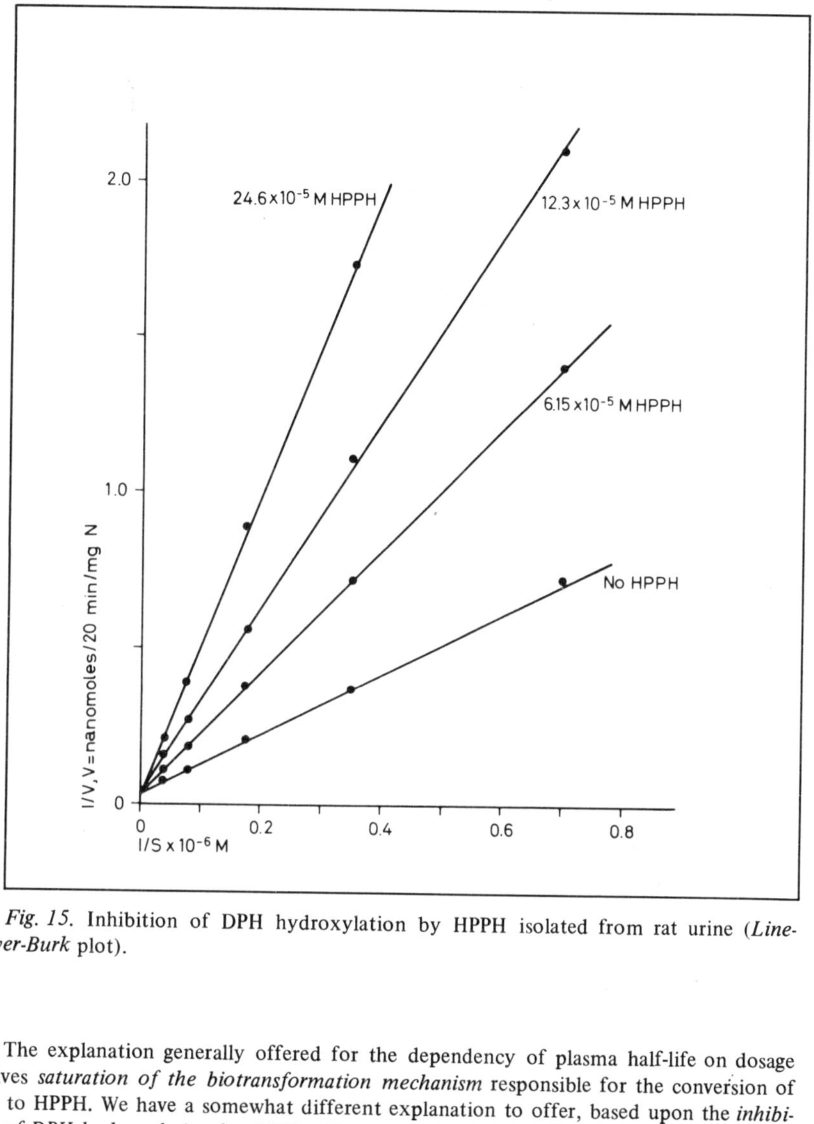

Fig. 15. Inhibition of DPH hydroxylation by HPPH isolated from rat urine (*Lineweaver-Burk* plot).

The explanation generally offered for the dependency of plasma half-life on dosage involves *saturation of the biotransformation mechanism* responsible for the conversion of DPH to HPPH. We have a somewhat different explanation to offer, based upon the *inhibition of DPH hydroxylation by HPPH* (19). Our first observations were made with 9,000 *g* supernate from rat liver homogenates, using DPH as a substrate and synthetic p-HPPH as an inhibitor. The results are shown in figure 14, in the form of a double reciprocal plot. Good inhibition of DPH hydroxylation was obtained. Since the synthetic HPPH is a racemic mixture, whereas the natural metabolite is optically active, the experiments were repeated with p-HPPH isolated from rat urine. The results shown in figure 15 clearly indicate that p-HPPH acts as a competitive inhibitor of DPH hydroxylation. The K_M value was 2.47×10^{-5} M, and V_{MAX} was 25 nmoles/mg N/20 min. The inhibitor constant K_i was

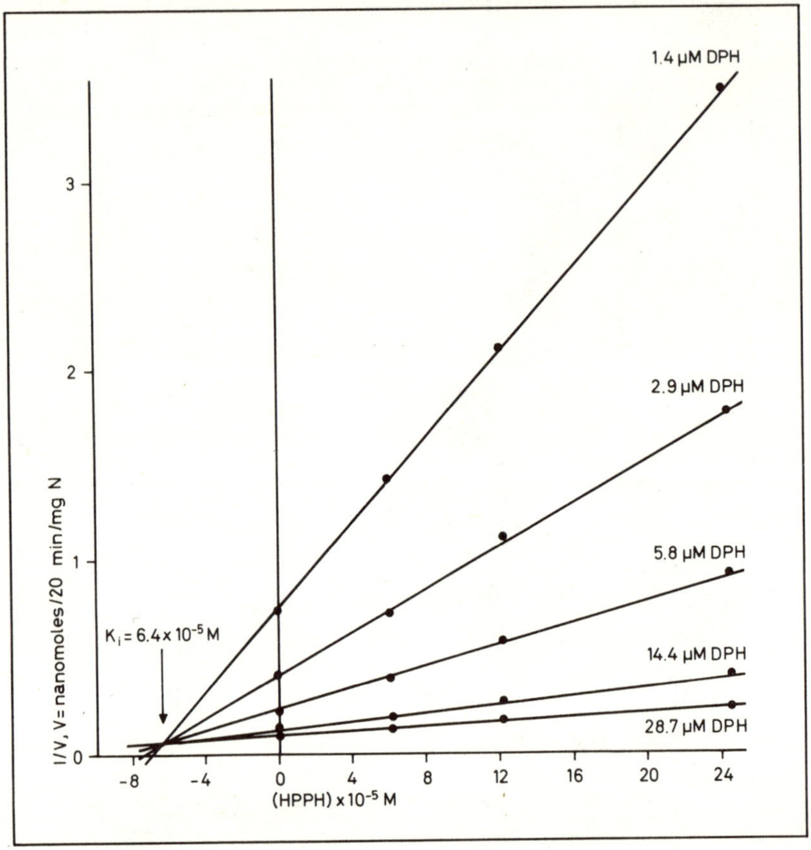

Fig. 16. Inhibition of DPH hydroxylation by HPPH isolated from rat urine (*Dixon* plot).

6.4×10^{-5} M, as indicated in figure 16. From these observations it appears that *the inhibition of DPH hydroxylation may be due to a feed-back mechanism in which the hydroxylated metabolite competes with DPH for a binding site on the enzyme complex.* This may offer a possible explanation for the dependency of DPH plasma half-life on dosage; it may also account for the great delay in the urinary excretion of HPPH noted earlier.

References

1 *Hall, D.G.:* Hearings before the Subcommittee on Monopoly, Select Committee on Small Business, US Senate, part 1, pp. 258–281 (Govnt. Printing Office, Washington, D.C. 1967).

2 *Eadie, M.J.; Sutherland, J.M., and Tyrer, J.H.:* Dilantin overdosage. Med. J. Austr. *ii:* 515 (1968).

3 *Rail, L.:* Dilantin overdosage. Med. J. Austr. *ii:* 339 (1968).
4 *Martin, C.M.; Rubin, M.; O'Malley, W.; Garaguai, V.F., and McCauley, C.E.:* Comparative physiological availability of 'brand' and 'generic' drugs in man: chloramphenicol, sulfisoxazole and diphenylhydantoin. Pharmacologist *10:* 167 (1968); see also J. amer. med. Ass. *205:* 23–30 (1968).
5 *Arnold, K.; Gerber, N., and Levy, G.:* Absorption and dissolution studies on sodium diphenylhydantoin capsules. Canad. J. Pharm. Sci. *5:* 89–92 (1970).
6 *Glazko, A.J.; Dill, W.A.; Drach, J.C., and Chang, T.:* Biological availability of drugs: evaluation from blood level and urinary excretion data. Symposium papers at 5th Nat. Meet. A.Ph.A. Acad. Pharm. Sci., pp. 326–343 (Amer. Pharmaceutical Ass., Washington, D.C. 1970).
7 *Glazko, A.J.; Chang, T.; Baukema, J.; Dill, W.A.; Goulet, J.R., and Buchanan, R.A.:* Metabolic disposition of diphenylhydantoin in normal human subjects following intravenous administration. Clin. Pharmacol. Ther. *10:* 498–504 (1969).
8 *Gerber, N.; Weller, W.L.; Lynn, R.; Rangno, R.E.; Sweetman, B.J., and Bush, M.T.:* Study of dose dependent metabolism of 5,5-diphenylhydantoin in the rat using new methodology for isolation and quantitation of metabolites *in vivo* and *in vitro.* J. Pharmacol. exp. Ther. *178:* 567–579 (1971).
9 *Butler, T.C.:* The metabolic conversion of 5,5-diphenylhydantoin to 5-(p-hydroxyphenyl)-5-phenylhydantoin. J. Pharmacol. exp. Ther. *119:* 1–11 (1957).
10 *Maynert, E.W.:* The metabolic fate of diphenylhydantoin in the dog, rat and man. J. Pharmacol. exp. Ther. *130:* 275–284 (1960).
11 *Chang, T. and Glazko, A.J.:* Quantitative assay of 5,5-diphenylhydantoin (DPH) and 5-(p-hydroxyphenyl)-5-phenylhydantoin by gas-liquid chromatography. J. Lab. clin. Med. *75:* 145–155 (1970).
12 *Dill, W.A.; Kazenko, A.; Wolf, L.M., and Glazko, A.J.:* Studies on 5,5-diphenylhydantoin (dilantin) in animals and man. J. Pharmacol. exp. Ther. *118:* 270–279 (1956).
13 *Remmer, H.; Hirschmann, J. und Greiner, I.:* Die Bedeutung von Kumulation und Elimination füf die Dosierung von Phenytoin (Diphenylhydantoin). Dtsch. med. Wschr. *94:* 1265–1272 (1969).
14 *Buchthal, F.; Svensmark, O., and Schiller, P.J.:* Clinical and encephalographic correlations with serum levels of diphenylhydantoin. Arch. Neurol., Chicago *2:* 624–630 (1960).
15 *Dayton, P.G.; Cucinell, S.A.; Weiss, M., and Perel, J.M.:* Dose-dependence of drug plasma level decline in dogs. J. Pharmacol. exp. Ther. *158:* 305–316 (1967).
16 *Arnold, K. and Gerber, N.:* The rate of decline of diphenylhydantoin in human plasma. Clin. Pharmacol. Ther. *11:* 121–134 (1970).
17 *Gerber, N. and Arnold, K.:* Studies on the metabolism of diphenylhydantoin in mice. J. Pharmacol. exp. Ther. *167:* 77–90 (1969).
18 *Buchanan, R.A.; Kinkel, A.W.; Goulet, J.R., and Smith, T.C.:* The metabolism of diphenylhydantoin (Dilantin) following once-daily administration. Neurology (Minneap.) *22:* 126–130 (1972).
19 *Borondy, P.; Chang, T., and Glazko, A.J.:* Inhibition of diphenylhydantoin hydroxylation by 5-(p-hydroxyphenyl)-5-phenylhydantoin (p-HPPH). Fed. Proc. *31:* 582 (1972).

Author's address: Dr. *Anthony J. Glazko,* Section Director, Chemical Pharmacology, Parke, Davis & Company, *Ann Arbor, MI 48106* (USA)

Biopharmaceutics of Nitrofurantoin

J.D. Conklin
Drug Distribution Unit, The Norwich Pharmacal Company, Norwich, N.Y.

Introduction

Biopharmaceutic investigations have rapidly become a principal center of activity in the pharmaceutical sciences. The increase in attention to this area is apparent from the number of conferences and symposia held and the many current textbooks and reports being published. Although often reiterated, it seems appropriate to consider again some of the basic factors which are involved in studying the biologic availability of drug formulations. Obviously, an adequate analytic method, with the desired sensitivity and specificity, is necessary to determine the drug or a related metabolite in various media. Drug absorption, distribution, metabolism, and elimination must be carefully investigated and examined for possible correlation with corresponding data on drug disintegration and dissolution. The controversy over using *in vitro* instead of *in vivo* methods to investigate the biologic availability of drug formulations continues without immediate apparent resolution. Unfortunately, difficulties occur with many drug formulations, in attempting to establish an *in vitro* to an *in vivo* correlation. At present, it appears that each drug formulation must be investigated as an independent entity. If studies are conducted in animals, consideration must be given to the differences that may exist between the species used and humans. Finally, it must not be overlooked that the ultimate purpose is to provide adequate drug efficacy through appropriate biologic availability.

History

The effectiveness of nitrofurantoin, 1-[(5-nitrofurfurylidene)amino]hydantoin, as a urinary tract antibacterial drug is well established. It is effective although blood drug levels seldom reach antibacterial concentrations. Instead, reliance is placed on bacteriostatic and bactericidal urine drug concentrations. Most outstanding during its widespread clinical use, has been the relatively limited incidence of serious side-effects and the minimal development of bacterial resistance. Since the first reports regarding its use appeared in 1952, many papers have provided information on nitrofurantoin. Occasionally, conflicting reports have appeared, as a result of additional knowledge subsequent to improvements in scientific techniques. The following presentation comprehensively represents the current biopharmaceutic information on nitrofurantoin, which is necessary for evaluating its biologic availability.

Nitrofurantoin Transfer

It is generally agreed that protein binding, degree of ionization, and lipid solubility are major factors regulating drug transfer. At pH 7.4, nitrofurantoin has a low lipid solubility, and about one half of the drug exists in its nonionized form. Accumulated values representing the binding of nitrofurantoin to plasma proteins vary widely. In essence, although a substantial amount of nitrofurantoin may be associated with plasma proteins shortly after the drug is administered, the binding appears to be readily reversible.

Absorption

Comparison of results obtained after peroral and intravenous administration of nitrofurantoin shows that perorally administered nitrofurantoin in a suitable dosage form is well absorbed. Nitrofurantoin absorption occurs primarily in the intestinal portion of the gastrointestinal tract, with little indication of any gastric absorption. Absorption from the small intestine is rapid and appears to follow the widely recognized pH-partition theory. Only limited drug absorption occurs when nitrofurantoin is administered rectally.

Distribution

During peroral therapeutic drug dosage, nitrofurantoin is seldom detectable in either plasma or whole blood. If detectable, the concentrations are low, usually less than 1 mg/l. However, nitrofurantoin levels about 3–5 times greater than this are usually found in these fluids when drug is administered intravenously or intramuscularly at clinical doses. Relatively equivalent amounts of nitrofurantoin are observed in plasma and whole blood.

Parenteral drug administration to man or animals at doses in excess of those used clinically results in detectable nitrofurantoin levels in several other body fluids. Concentrations of nitrofurantoin in aqueous humor, cerebrospinal fluid and prostatic fluid are considerably lower than those noted in corresponding blood specimens. Thoracic and renal lymph levels of nitrofurantoin closely approximate those concurrently found in blood. The levels of nitrofurantoin noted in bile and urine are greatly in excess of the related blood drug concentrations.

Studies with ^{14}C-nitrofurantoin have shown levels of radioactivity in most mammalian tissues, without any apparent preferential depots. Only traces of nitrofurantoin are found in the liver and kidney shortly after intravenous drug administration.

Elimination

Usually, large amounts of nitrofurantoin are recovered from the excretory fluids, bile and urine, after either peroral or parenteral drug administration. Detectable fecal drug levels are only encountered occasionally.

Nitrofurantoin is excreted in the kidney by glomerular filtration and is both secreted and reabsorbed in the tubules. Nitrofurantoin clearance in the kidney is handled by a weak-acid transport system which is influenced by pH. Under acid conditions, tubular reabsorption is increased, presumably resulting in higher kidney tissue drug levels. Alkaline conditions reduce this effect, evidently yielding greater nitrofurantoin concentrations in urine. During renal impairment, nitrofurantoin urinary excretion is significantly decreased.

It appears that nitrofurantoin transfer through the liver is also handled by a weak-acid transport system. A dose-related increase in bile flow, which is primarily hydrocholeretic in nature, has been observed in dogs. Some of the drug excreted in dog bile is reabsorbed and subjected to enterohepatic recirculation.

Most mammalian tissues are capable of readily destroying nitrofurantoin. Intestinal contents, containing bacteria, enzymes, and feces, must be considered as an additional factor in nitrofurantoin destruction. It is, therefore, assumed that a substantial amount of nitrofurantoin is also eliminated by enzymatic degradation.

Pharmacokinetics

The maximum nitrofurantoin blood concentration obtained immediately after intravenous drug administration is only about one fifth of the level anticipated if the total dose was confined to only the blood volume. This suggests that nitrofurantoin is readily distributed into the extracellular and intracellular compartments. The transfer of nitrofurantoin across body membranes apparently occurs by diffusion, with the exception of the active drug secretion in the kidney-tubule and biliary drug transport.

Nitrofurantoin has a half-life in blood or plasma of about 30 min or less, and the disappearance apparently follows first-order kinetics. In conjunction with this disappearance, nitrofurantoin is rapidly excreted in both bile and urine. Also, there is little evidence for any prolonged binding of nitrofurantoin to either plasma proteins or tissues. At present, a one-compartment model appears to be most appropriate for describing the kinetics involved in nitrofurantoin absorption and excretion.

The results presented show that nitrofurantoin is readily absorbed and quickly distributed into most body fluids, and that biliary and urinary excretion of unchanged nitrofurantoin and enzymatic degradation are the primary means of elimination. These observations explain, at least partially, why significant biologic drug residues have not been encountered with nitrofurantoin under clinical conditions.

Bioavailability

Since relatively low nitrofurantoin blood levels are encountered after peroral drug administration, it is usually necessary to use nitrofurantoin urinary excretion as a parameter for evaluating the biologic availability of nitrofurantoin formulations. Studies conducted with intravenously administered drug establish that the drug level in both blood and urine is proportional to dose, and that nitrofurantoin urinary excretion may be used as a reliable indicator for the *in vivo* absorption of nitrofurantoin. Results obtained from numerous studies show that similarities or differences between nitrofurantoin formulations are readily discernible using this approach.

Nitrofurantoin urinary drug recoveries obtained in humans after peroral and intravenous clinical doses establish that the Eaton nitrofurantoin tablet and Eaton nitrofurantoin oral suspension are well absorbed. Although the suspension is more readily available initially than the tablet, both formulations ultimately yield equivalent biologic availability. A number of patients have experienced nausea or emesis with these formulations to the extent that effective nitrofurantoin medication was not administered. The development of the Eaton nitrofurantoin macrocrystals provided a means of reducing the incidence of this gastrointestinal intolerance to nitrofurantoin. Essentially, the formulation consists of encapsulated nitrofurantoin macrocrystals which are better tolerated gastrointestinally and also absorbed sufficiently to achieve effective therapy.

The majority of the accumulated information on the availability of Eaton nitrofurantoin formulations has been obtained using *in vivo* methods. Information regarding some of the *in vitro* characteristics of these formulations is stipulated in the USP.

At this time, it is appropriate to consider an aspect which is sometimes neglected during the evaluation of accumulated information on the availability of certain drug formulations. Unfortunately, several of the approaches and techniques now used in drug formulation availability investigations were not available when nitrofurantoin was introduced for clinical use. In addition, if clinical results show that a drug formulation is effective, then there is little practical reason for conducting additional availability studies at a later date with newly-developed techniques. As a result of this, little information has been obtained on possible correlations between *in vitro* and *in vivo* results concerning the availability of Eaton nitrofurantoin formulations. Recently, a few reports concerning such correlations with various nitrofurantoin formulations have been presented. Unfortunately, the data are not sufficient to establish completely a reliable correlation between the two approaches. However, there is the indication of a general trend, in that long drug formulation disintegration and dissolution times are often related to limited biologic availability.

Conclusion

Nitrofurantoin is another drug whose biologic availability and subsequent therapeutic properties are susceptible to the influence of formulation variations. Relative to this, the following aspects are reiterated concerning the biopharmaceutics of nitrofurantoin. Urinary drug excretion, instead of blood drug levels, must be utilized to investigate nitrofurantoin biologic availability. It also appears, at present, that the most reliable means for evaluating the biologic availability of nitrofurantoin formulations is by an *in vivo* method. Finally, consideration must be given to examining the relationship of this biologic availability to efficacy.

I sincerely hope that some of the information I have presented on nitrofurantoin will assist you in dealing with the problems we all face today in providing drug formulations with appropriate biologic availability, which will yield adequate efficacy with minimal side-effects.

Author's address: Dr. *John D. Conklin*, Senior Scientist, Drug Distribution Unit, The Norwich Pharmacal Company, 17 Eaton Avenue, *Norwich, NY 13815* (USA)

Sodium Warfarin

R.A. O'Reilly
Department of Medicine, Santa Clara Valley Medical Center, San Jose, Calif.

As perhaps the only practicing clinician on this program, it may be my responsibility to define bioavailability more in terms of the patient we all serve. The brochure for this conference defines bioavailability in pharmacokinetic terms, the appearance of drug in the general circulation. I shall additionally define bioavailability in pharmacodynamic terms, the biologic effect in the patient, and observe the correlation of these two parameters of drug metabolism. Sodium warfarin is an ideal agent for this challenge because of the ease in quantifying both the anticoagulant effect and the drug itself in man.

To quickly review some of the known chemical and pharmacological facts about sodium warfarin, the structural formula is shown in figure 1. The two parts of the molecule are the 4-hydroxycoumarin moiety on the left and the acetonylbenzyl side-chain on the right. The intact coumarin moiety is the more important for anticoagulant effect as the

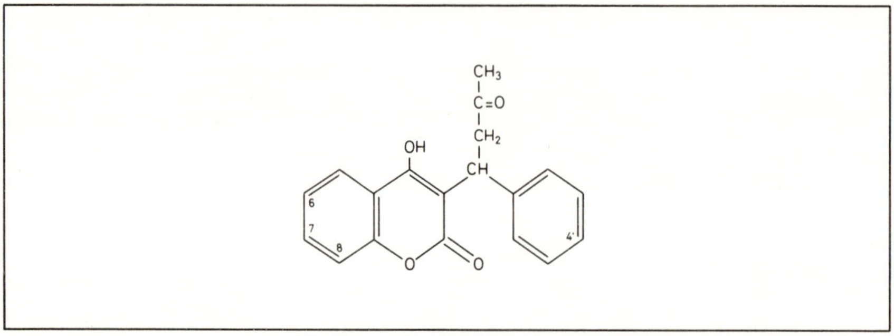

Fig. 1. Structural formula of sodium warfarin (8).

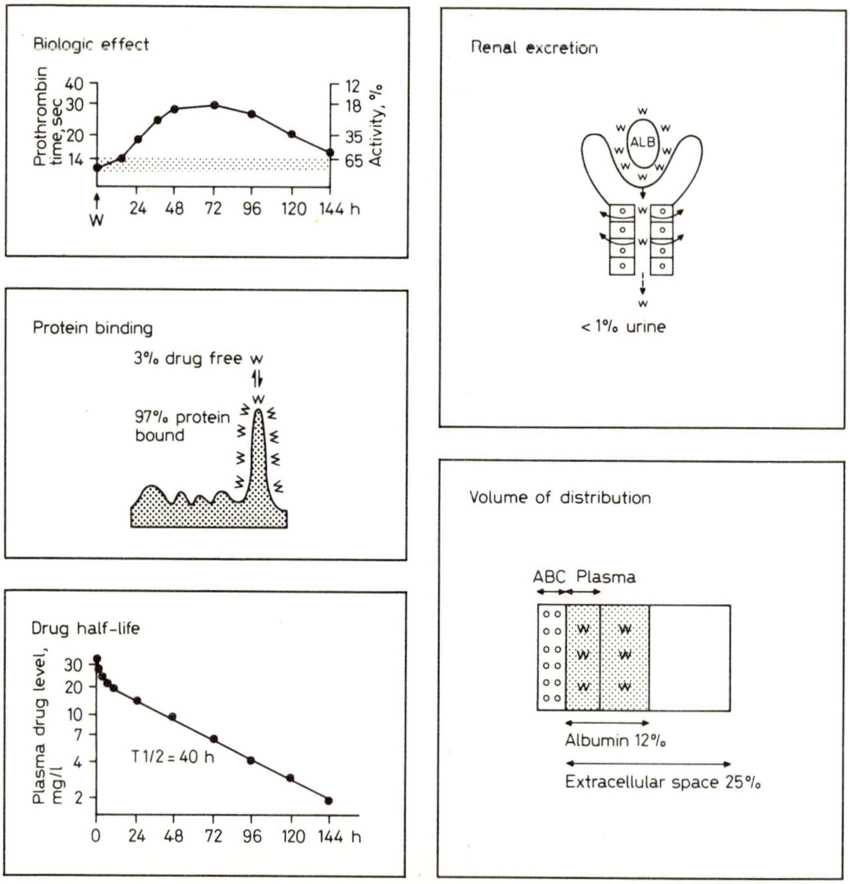

Fig. 2. Some aspects of clinical pharmacology of warfarin (4).

introduction of any group, particularly hydroxyl groups by metabolism, results in complete loss of biologic activity. The enol function af the 4-position allows the manufacture of the sodium salt.

Figure 2 summarizes some aspects of the clinical pharmacology of warfarin. Many of the pharmacologic details may result from its extensive binding to plasma albumin: the long half-life in plasma (40 h), the long anticoagulant effect (7–10 days), the lack of renal excretion of unchanged drug, the absence of drug in red blood cells or cerebrospinal fluid, and a volume of distribution the size of the albumin space.

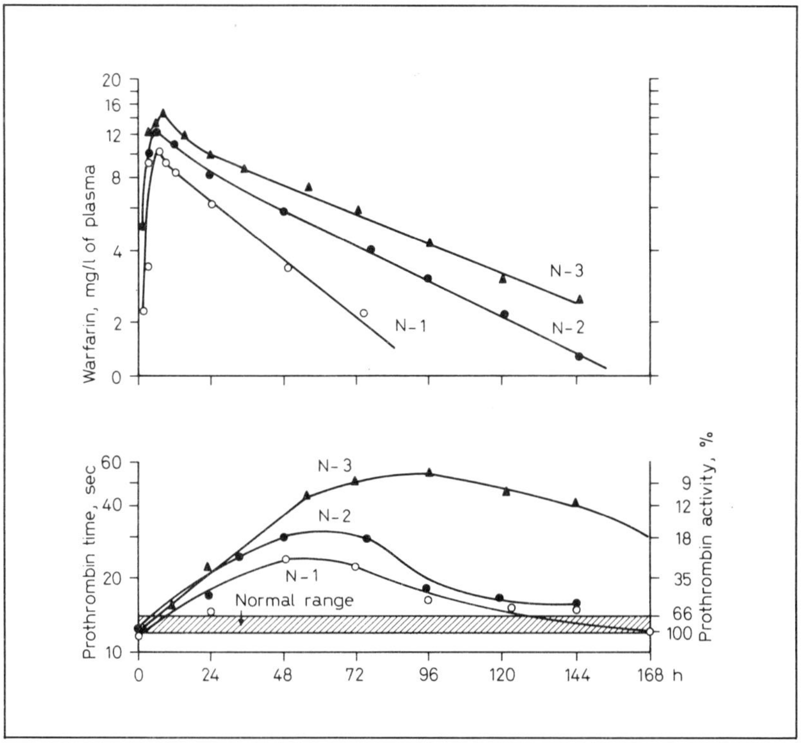

Fig. 3. Correlation of blood levels of drug and anticoagulant effect in three normal subjects (7).

Figure 3 shows the correlation of the blood levels of drug and the anticoagulant effect in three normal subjects. The higher the drug levels or the more prolonged the half-life of warfarin, the greater the area under the curve for the anticoagulant effect. This correlation is found not only in different individuals but in the same individual when the pharmacokinetics of warfarin are altered by other drugs.

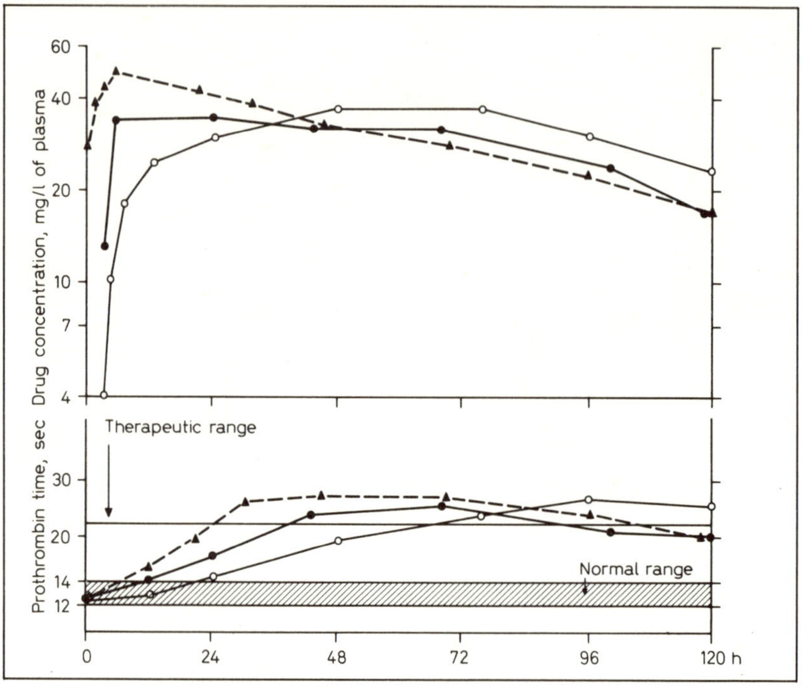

Fig. 4. Effect of dose form on the bioavailability of another oral anticoagulant, bishydroxycoumarin (subject N-2). ○ = Tablet 600 mg; ● = powder 600 mg; ▲ = solution 550 mg (5).

Figure 4 illustrates the effect of dose form on the bioavailability of another oral anticoagulant, bishydroxycoumarin, in one normal subject. Note the marked effect of the powder and solution forms not only on the earlier appearance of the drug in plasma but also on the earlier appearance of a significant anticoagulant effect – from 72 h for tablet form to 24 h for the solution form – a 3-fold difference. These data indicate the rate-limiting effect of the dissolution step with a drug that has poor aqueous solubility.

Figure 5 astounded the late Dr. *Eino Nelson* when he first saw it. On comparison of tablets of sodium warfarin (the USP form) with plain warfarin or warfarin free acid (the rodenticidal form), both the drug levels and the significant anticoagulant effect appeared earlier with the warfarin acid.

Fig. 5. Comparative gastrointestinal absorption of warfarin tablets and solution (subject N-2). 100 mg of drug *per os.* ▲ = Warfarin Na tablets; ● = warfarin acid tablets; ○ = warfarin Na solution (5).

Fig. 6. Semilogarithmic plot of percent warfarin undissolved from several tablet formulations versus time. The medium used was distilled water (10).

Fig. 7. Apparent first-order dissolution of warfarin preparations A and D. Conditions: 30 min dissolution in 0.1 N HCl, then dissolution in the medium brought to pH 7.4 by adding tris(hydroxymethyl) aminomethane (10).

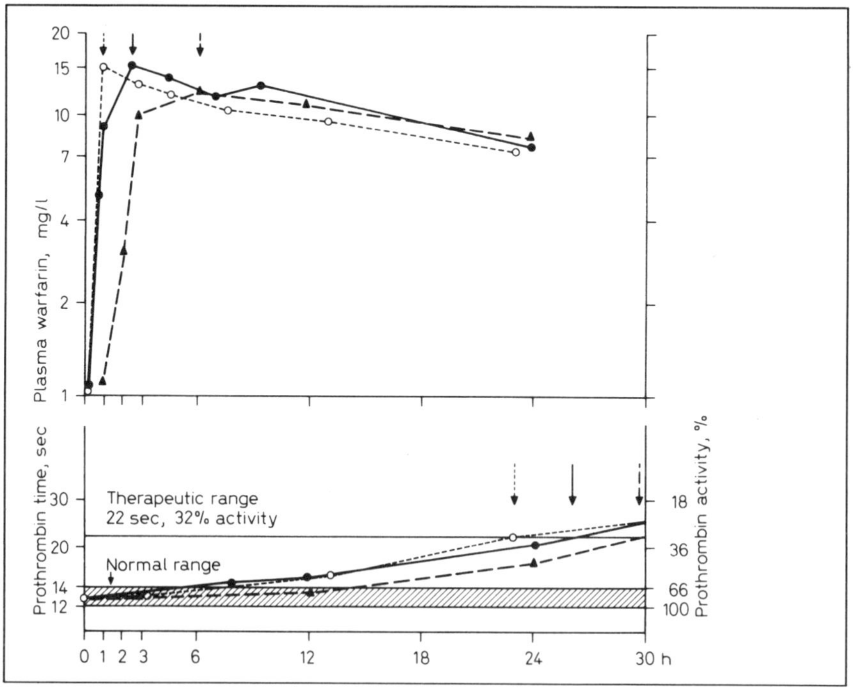
Plasma warfarin, mg/l
Prothrombin time, sec
Prothrombin activity, %
Therapeutic range
22 sec, 32% activity
Normal range
0 1 2 3 6 12 18 24 30 h

5

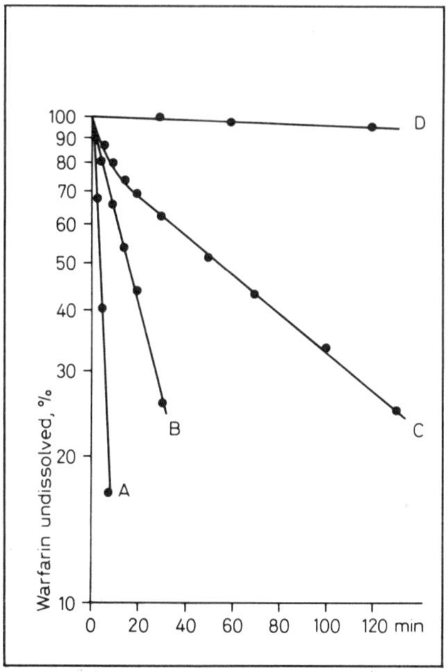
Warfarin undissolved, %
A
B
C
D
0 20 40 60 80 100 120 min

6

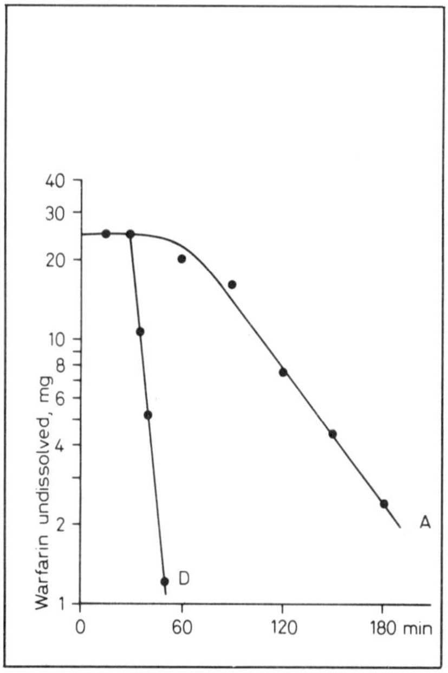
Warfarin undissolved, mg
A
D
0 60 120 180 min

7

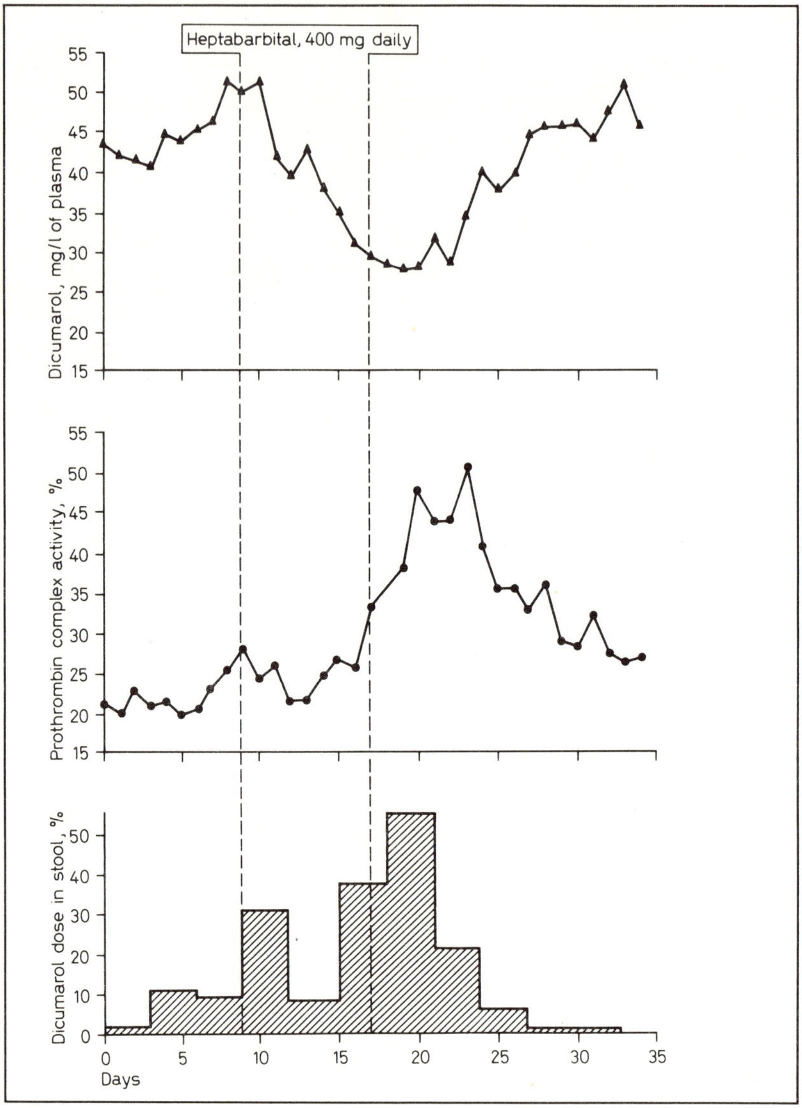

8

Fig. 8. Alteration of the physiologic availability by another drug (2).

Fig. 9. Effect of administration of phenylbutazone on the prothrombin response and on the plasma level and disappearance rate of warfarin in a normal subject (N-22). Phenylbutazone, 600 mg/day, was given by mouth for 3 days before and for the duration of the experiment after administration of a standard dose of warfarin, 1.5 mg/kg of body weight, given orally. • = With phenylbutazone; ○ = without phenylbutazone (6).

Fig. 10. Phenylbutazone (100 mg/l) successfully competing with warfarin (2–200 mg/l) for binding sites on plasma albumin (0.4 %). • = present; ○ = absent.

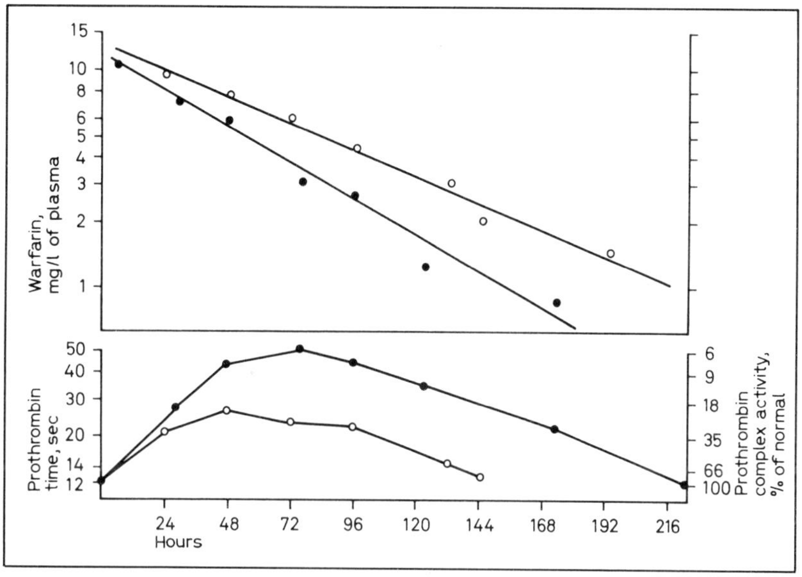
Warfarin, mg/l of plasma
15
10
8
6
5
4
3
2
1
Prothrombin time, sec
50
40
30
20
14
12
Prothrombin complex activity, % of normal
6
9
18
35
66
100
24
48
72
96
120
144
168
192
216
Hours

9

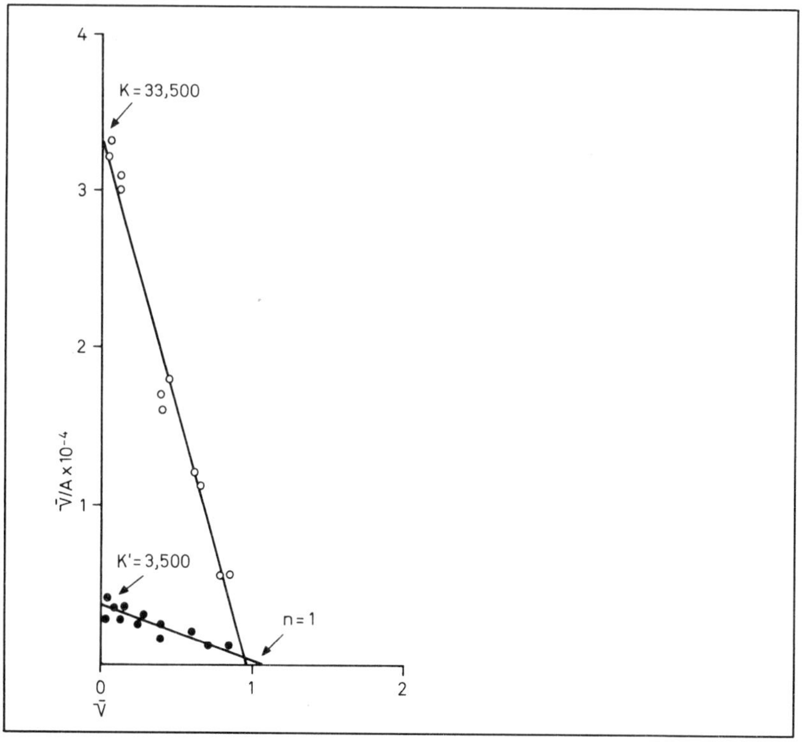
K = 33,500
K' = 3,500
n = 1
$\bar{\nu}$/A x 10^{-4}
4
3
2
1
0
1
2
$\bar{\nu}$

10

Figure 6 shows the dissolution-rate studies on tablets of sodium warfarin (preparations A, B, and C) and of warfarin acid (preparation D) in distilled water. The warfarin acid appears to have a hopelessly long dissolution rate. Figure 7 shows the dissolution rate of tablet A (sodium warfarin) and tablet D (warfarin acid) in buffer at pH 7.4 after a 30-min exposure to 0.1 N hydrochloric acid. The dissolution rates under these conditions show an excellent correlation with the surprisingly rapid absorption of the warfarin acid tablets. This study also underscores the need for the formulation of compressed tablets in which the release of the active ingredient is not a sensitive function of pH in the physiologic range.

Figure 8 shows how one drug can alter the physiologic availability of another drug. It shows that, in addition to its traditional role of induction of hepatic enzymes, barbiturate reduces the absorption of bishydroxycoumarin as the greatly increased quantity of unchanged bishydroxycoumarin in stool was seen only after its oral administration.

Figure 9 shows how the amount of drug entering the circulation can be misleading. Here is the well-known *potentiation* of anticoagulant effect by phenylbutazone in man, yet the blood levels of warfarin are actually *lessened* by the second drug.

In figure 10 this Scatchard plot shows that phenylbutazone successfully competes with warfarin for binding sites on plasma albumin and perhaps makes more free warfarin available to its sites of biologic effect and metabolism.

Figure 11 shows another example of misinformation when one measures only drug levels, this time a pharmacogenetic example as illustrated by the propositus of the first reported kindred with hereditary resistance to oral anticoagulants. Here the bioavailability of drug in plasma is perfectly normal yet the biologic effect is almost nil.

Figure 12 shows yet another example of misinformation when one measures only drug levels in blood, this time the result of the presence of large amounts of vitamin K, the specific antidote for oral anticoagulants. Again, the bioavailability of drug is perfectly normal with vitamin K, but the medicinal power of the anticoagulant drug has been markedly reduced.

In conclusion, I would like to say that studies on the bioavailability of drugs are more powerful when their pharmacokinetic and pharmacodynamic aspects can be quantitated and correlated in man. This approach is implicit in the stated goals of the first USP Convention of 1820: 'It is the object of a pharmacopeia to select from among substances which possess medicinal power those the utility of which is best understood ... [and] to form from them preparations and compositions in which their powers may be exerted to the greatest advantage.' I submit to you that everyone at this conference believes in medicinal power. When the appropriate committee eventually writes the standards for the physiologic availability of drugs, they must look beyond the pharmaceutical curtain and consider not only the 'pill' but also the patient. The standards for the bioavailability of drugs must consider the factors that affect medicinal power in drug recipients. These factors include age (both infants and the elderly), disease states (particularly gastrointestinal, hepatic, and renal), pregnancy, other drugs, and the genetic pool of the recipients.

Fig. 11. Showing an example of misinformation when one measures only drug levels (warfarin orally, 1.5 mg/kg), this time a pharmacogenetic example as illustrated by the propositus of the first reported kindred with hereditary resistance to oral anticoagulants. Here the bioavailability of drug in plasma is perfectly normal yet the biologic effect is almost nil.

Fig. 12. Warfarin 1.5 mg/kg orally (subject N-4). ● = Alone; ○ = with vitamin K, 5 mg/8 h/4 days until time 0 (8). The blood levels of warfarin are unaltered by the vitamin K, but the prothrombin time response has been markedly reduced.

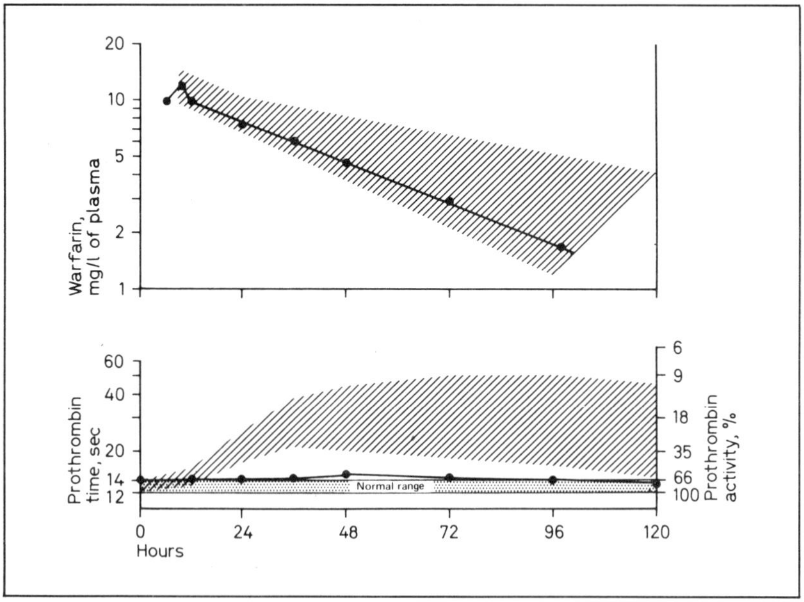
20
10
5
2
1
Warfarin, mg/l of plasma
60
40
20
14
12
Prothrombin time, sec
6
9
18
35
66
100
Prothrombin activity, %
Normal range
0
24
48
72
96
120
Hours

11

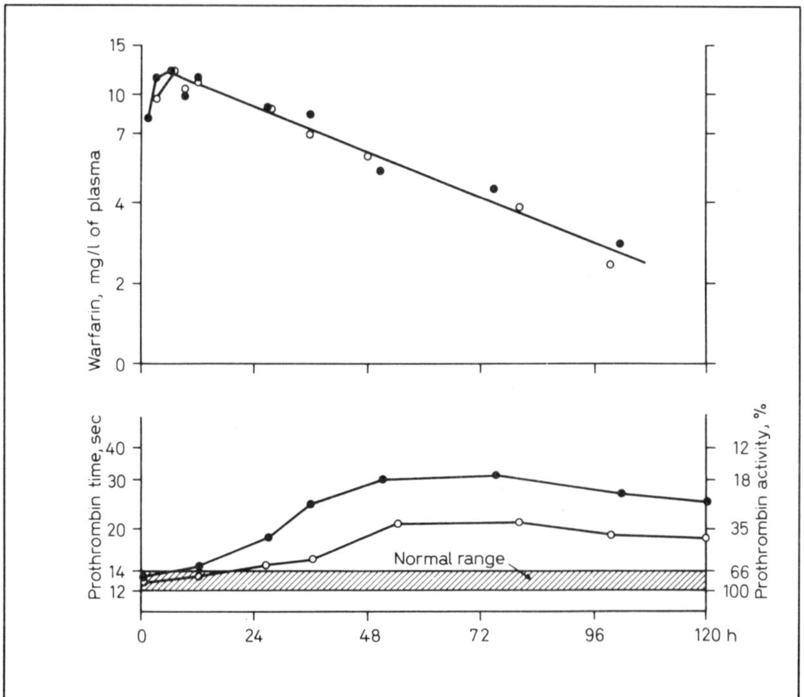
15
10
7
4
2
0
Warfarin, mg/l of plasma
40
30
20
14
12
Prothrombin time, sec
12
18
35
66
100
Prothrombin activity, %
Normal range
0
24
48
72
96
120 h

12

References

1 *Aggeler, P.M. et al.:* New Engl. J. Med. *276:* 496 (1967).
2 *Aggeler, P.M. and O'Reilly, R.A.:* J. Lab. clin. Med. *74:* 229 (1969).
3 *O'Reilly, R.A.:* J. clin. Invest. *48:* 193 (1969).
4 *O'Reilly, R.A.:* Clinical pharmacology of anticoagulant therapy; in Science and practice of clinical medicine (Grune & Stratton, New York, in press).
5 *O'Reilly, R.A. and Aggeler, P.M.:* Thromb. Diath. haemorrh. *11:* 1 (1964).
6 *O'Reilly, R.A. and Aggeler, P.M.:* Proc. Soc. exp. Biol. Med. *128:* 1280 (1968).
7 *O'Reilly, R.A. et al.:* Thromb. Diath. haemorrh. *8:* 82 (1962).
8 *O'Reilly, R.A. et al.:* J. clin. Invest. *42:* 1542 (1963).
9 *O'Reilly, R.A. et al.:* Ann. N.Y. Acad. Sci. *151:* 913 (1968).
10 *O'Reilly, R.A.; Nelson, E., and Levy, G.:* J. pharm. Sci. *55:* 435 (1966).

Author's address: Prof. *Robert A. O'Reilly,* Chairman, Department of Medicine, Santa Clara Valley Medical Center, 751 So. Bascom Ave, *San Jose, CA 95128* (USA)

Canadian Experience

D. Cook

Pharmaceutical Chemistry Division, Food and Drug Directorate, Department of National Health and Welfare, Ottawa, Ont.

I am pleased to have this opportunity to describe to you some of the experiences we have had at the Canadian Food and Drug Directorate in dealing with the question of bioavailability of solid oral dosage forms.

It would be appropriate first of all to discuss what we did both in the early days in the mid-fifties and early sixties, and latterly in the stepped-up program of investigation, and follow this by an estimate of the significance of the results generated and of the relationship between these measurements and *in vitro* parameters such as dissolution rate and disintegration time.

The concept of bioavailability (which was known in the late forties as physiological availability) (1) arose out of comparisons of the physiological effects produced by commercial dosage forms and a reference substance, usually chosen so that its formulation had no effect upon the rate of uptake and utilization of the active ingredient.

Much of the earlier work was done using vitamin preparations and there were clear demonstrations of the inhibition, by the design of the dosage form, of the utilization of the active ingredient. Some of these investigations involved rather unusual dosage forms: those designed for special release properties, or with unusual coatings for special purposes.

It will be clear that there are two possible conditions under which bioavailability variations become significant. The first of these is when across a spectrum of manufactured products there are wide variations in bioavailability so that changing from one product to another might cause differences in therapeutic effect.

The second would be the planned change in a drug product formulation by a product development group, without checking the reformulated product *in vivo.* Apparently this occurred recently with the anticoagulants and hypoglycemic agents. It will also be clear that there are two directions in which biological availability can change. Firstly, bioavailability can decrease with a resultant potential lack of therapeutic effect, or it can increase with the development of adverse reactions or toxicity or excessive action over and above that required.

From the viewpoint of the consumer one of the first things we want to ensure is protection against some dosage form being ineffective, either through ignorance or error, because the proportion of the dose absorbed is so low as to elicit no pharmacologic effect. The second is to protect against a variation which delivers much more drug when compared to an accepted norm, and which may be associated with toxic reactions.

The third objective is to generate an information system so that for those critical drugs we can define precisely what absorption rate, peak height, peak time, and excretion curve, is necessary to get the optimum value from a dosage form. We are still asking those questions that *Lasagna* put so pointedly in Ottawa in 1969 (2).

While we share the same dilemma with the United States Pharmacopeia and the Drug Research Board of not knowing, for most drugs, what blood level is effective for a particular indication, we are taking steps to ensure the use of products with a certain level of acceptable bioavailability. This has not appeared in a regulation as yet, but is a device whereby products which have been tested in a study are not included in certain lists if they have failed to meet this particular level (3).

To retreat a little in time and give some details of the developments leading up to this concept would be appropriate.

In 1967 a Parliamentary Committee of the Canadian House of Commons under the chairmanship of Dr. *H.C. Harley* was instituted with terms of reference empowering it to look into 'drug costs and drug prices'. Countless briefs and opinions were heard, and eventually a series of recommendations ensued from this committee. One of these was fairly generally approved, and is as follows (4):

That the Food and Drug Directorate publish not less than once a month an informative bulletin containing: (a) generic name of the drug; (b) names of all manufacturers of the drug, and brand names of the above drug; (c) comparative costs and clinical equivalency of the above drugs; (d) therapeutic action of drug; (e) side effects of drug, contraindications and toxicity; (f) last assay for each company's product, of content and availability of active ingredient, solubility and disintegration, and (g) any problems with any company's product – toxicity, impurity, seizures, court actions, failure to meet standards, etc.

This recommendation was accepted by FDD in 1969 and plans were implemented to publish at regular intervals the information that Dr. *Harley* thought members of the health professions were lacking. These plans called for the generation of analytical data on the *in vitro* aspects of drug quality. They also called for a program of measuring bioavailability data in humans, not for selected products of a certain drug, but for all commercially available products of (a certain strength of) that drug.

Certain decisions had to be made very early in this implementation. The question of patients or non-patients had to be answered. For reasons familiar to all we decided to choose healthy, normal public servants. Their response has been one of the most encouraging features of the whole program and we acknowledge a debt of gratitude to them.

The question of what comparison dosage form should be used to assess bioavailability, defined for blood level studies as AUC (area under blood level-time curve) test product to AUC reference product, or for urinary excretion studies, as ratio of amount excreted test product to reference product, was solved by selecting the innovators product. This provides the link to a product that has been through the new drug approval procedures that a physician would be expected to want. (Where no unequivocal innovator can be identified a non-commercial reference substance is chosen.)

The criteria by which we chose the drug to be studied were made clear from the outset and included medical purpose, criticality of dose, available methodology, hazards to volunteers, cost/benefit ratios, and known problems with variation in bioavailability. A committee on human studies is asked to comment on all protocols for human investigations and a group of statistical scientists furnishes advice on design of the protocol and patterns of product administration. To these two groups of people we owe a great deal: without them we could not let one drop of blood flow, nor collect one fluid ounce of urine.

Another consideration in the overall development of the bioavailability study was the desirability of establishing correlations between the *in vivo* results and some physicochemical parameter which would serve as a marker of predictive value in humans, and would be cheap and easy to perform. An FDD representative joined in most of the committee meetings of the original USP/NF Joint Panel on Physiological Availability, and stressed the value of such *in vivo/in vitro* correlations.

For the benefit of those unfamiliar with Canadian legislation a variety of books of drug standards are official in Canada. These reflect our cultural background and, therefore, should include the Pharmacopée Française and the British Pharmacopoeia and British Pharmaceutical Codex. They also reflect our trading habits, and thus include the United States Pharmacopeia and the National Formulary.

Because of this multiplicity of standards it is not sufficient to say we approve the dissolution test in the United States Pharmacopeia for Hydrochlorothiazide, or in the National Formulary for Methylprednisolone for example. A manufacturer may elect to choose a standard from the British Pharmacopoeia or the British Pharmaceutical Codex, or the Codex Français, and thereby avoid, if he so wishes, the provisions of the North American Pharmacopeia. This situation might be especially true in the case of a manufacturer who had evidence of the acceptable bioavailability of his product but an unsatisfactory dissolution rate parameter.

The purpose of this meeting is to come to grips with the problem of defining adequate levels of drug bioavailability. Some brief summary of our experience may be helpful at this stage. In the pilot studies that characterized some earlier work there were examples of inadequacies in some dosage forms. Among these might be mentioned PAS, various vitamins, iron salts, sulfa drugs. Many of these were associated with unusual coatings, special release forms, etc.

In the recent across-the-board surveys where specific collections were taken at the manufacturing level our recent experience has been good.

Nitrofurantoin Study (Blood Level and Urinary Excretion) (5)

18 commercial formulations were tested. The strength used for this survey tablets of 100 mg. A design based on three 7 × 7 Latin squares was followed. Urinary excretion of the unchanged drug was determined at 1, 2, 3, 4, 5, 6, 8 and 10 h, but in one of the groups, in addition, blood samples (microlance finger puncture) were taken at $^1/_2$, $^3/_4$, 1, 1$^1/_2$, 2, 2$^1/_2$, 3, 4 and 6 h, measuring unchanged drug. A preliminary 100-mg ingestion of the standard (< 200 mesh in gelatin capsule) was taken by all volunteers in order to choose homogeneous groups for each Latin square.

The assay techniques described by *Conklin and Hollifield* (6) formed the basis of the method for drug determination. The blood level and excretion data are summarized as follows: peak blood level (6 dosage forms) 0.8–1.6 μg/ml; time to reach peak blood level 1.5–1.8 h; time to reach 30 μg/ml in urine 0.6–2.7 h; bioavailability (control) 67–109 %

Dissolution rate data: USP XVIII ($^{t}60$) 15 to 267 ($^{t}20$ value) min; resin kettle pH 7.2 phosphate buffer ($^{t}50$) 7 to > 136 min; stationary basket gastric fluid ($^{t}50$) 5 to > 85 min; stationary basket intestinal fluid ($^{t}50$) 4 to > 131 min.

Bioavailability/dissolution rate correlations were attempted between (a) the USP XVIII test, $^{t}60$ value and (i) 3-hour excretion; (ii) bioavailability; (iii) time to reach 30 μg/ml urine; (iv) time to peak blood level, and (b) amount dissolved in first hour versus amount excreted in first hour. In the best correlation (b) the value of $100r^2$ (r = correlation coefficient) was only 68, when a value of 90–100 is required for predictive purposes (7).

Phenylbutazone (Pilot Study only, Blood Level) (8)

Ten subjects used 9 brands of the 30 or so brands commercially available in Canada. A 5 × 5 Latin square with 5 products was used for the first group followed by 4 brands and one control suspension: all 5 volunteers taking the same brand at the same time. Two weeks elapsed between administrations. 2 × 100 mg was the regular test dose, and 200 mg phenylbutazone solution (pH, 7.4, 2.5 % w/v lactose) was the control. Blood samples were taken at 2, 4, 6, 8, 12, 24 and 48 h.

The blood level data are summarized as follows: Peak blood level 20.8–37 μg/ml; time to reach peak blood level 2.4–8.4 h; bioavailability (control) 61.3–104 %.

Dissolution rate data (intestinal fluid, pH 7.4). Stationary basket ($^{t}50$) 28.1–994.6 min; FDD disintegration ($^{t}50$) (5 dosage forms) 25.5–380.1 min; resin kettle ($^{t}50$) 32.1–498 min; *Levy* beaker ($^{t}50$) 25.6–665.3 min.

Subsequent dissolution tests were carried out on the same dosage forms used in the *in vivo* study using the conditions newly outlined in the first supplement to USP XVIII. No correlation was established with the original tests, and the latest USP XVIII first supplement test would class as unsatisfactory several products of satisfactory bioavailability.

Sulfamethizole (Blood Level and Urinary Excretion) (9)

Three different manufacturers products were tested, the dose ingested being 500 mg, taken $1\frac{1}{2}$ h after a standard breakfast. Blood was collected at $\frac{1}{2}$, $\frac{3}{4}$, 1, $1\frac{1}{2}$, $2\frac{1}{2}$, 4 and 6 h, and urine at 1, 2, 3, 5, 7, 10, 14 and 24 h. Unchanged sulfamethizole and total sulfamethizole in blood, and total sulfamethizole in urine were determined by the *Bratton-Marshall* procedure. The control was a suspension of 500 mg of known particle size range in 200 ml water. A 5 × 5 Latin square with weekly intervals between dosing was followed.

The blood level and urinary excretion data are summarized as follows: Peak blood level 17.8–21.7 μg/ml; time to reach peak blood level 1.5–2.6 h; $t\frac{1}{2}$ absorption 0.38–0.66 h; $t\frac{1}{2}$ elimination 1.24–1.37 h; bioavailability (blood level data) 96.5–110 %; bioavailability (urinary excretion data) 92–109 %.

Hydrochlorothiazide (Urinary Excretion Study) (10)

36 products were tested in 4 10 × 10 Latin squares. The 50-mg strength was used. A control dose of a 50-mg suspension in 200 ml water was used. An adequate programmed water intake was scheduled and a standard breakfast taken $1\frac{1}{2}$ h before ingestion of the dosage form. One week elapsed between treatments. Urine collections were made at 1, 2, 3,

4, 5, 8, 11, 14 and 24 h. Unchanged drug in urine (60 %) was assayed by the method of *Sheppard et al.*

The bioavailability of these products ranged from 88–113 %, and the dissolution rate data using the USP XVIII conditions gave t_{60} values of from 1.5–195 min. The limit quoted is 60 % dissolved in not more than 30 min.

Chlorothiazide (Urinary Excretion) (10)

A 5 × 5 Latin square design was used to examine 4 products (500 mg strength), and a control suspension of 500 mg chlorothiazide in water was used. Urine collections were made at 0, 1, 2, 3, 4, 5, 8, 11, 14 and 24 h. A standard breakfast was taken 1½ h prior to ingestion. Programmed intake of water was maintained during day 1.

Acetaminophen (Blood Level and Urinary Excretion) (11)

Nine products and a standard were taken by 10 volunteers in a 10 × 10 Latin square with weekly intervals between ingestions of 1 g of drug; the control was 1 g pure drug in 100 ml H_2O. Programmed water intake was observed. Blood samples were taken at ⅓, ⅔, 1, 1½, 2, 4 and 6 h. Urine samples were taken at 1, 1½, 2, 2½, 3, 4, 5, 8, 11, 14 and 24 h.

The blood level and urinary excretion data are summarized as follows: Peak blood levels 15.3–20.6 μg/ml; time to reach peak 55–96 min; time to reach 10 μg/ml 24.2–59.7 min; time at 10 μg/ml 101–175 min; bioavailability (blood level data, free acetaminophen) 78.4–102.7 %; bioavailability (urinary excretion data, total, acetaminophen and conjugates) 85.3–97.7 %.

Dissolution rate data obtained were as follows: USP XVIII (gastric buffer, T_{50}) 1–20 min; resin kettle (gastric buffer, T_{50}) 1–30.5 min; stationary basket (gastric buffer, T_{50}) 4–36 min; stationary basket (intestinal buffer, T_{50}) 1–106 min; resin kettle (intestinal buffer, T_{50}) 1–126 min.

None of the studies that we have done so far with any dissolution apparatus, have given us confidence that we have a cheap, simple, *in vitro* test of dissolution that would be predictive of the physiological response in man. Some parameters have come close but lack that refinement that is considered necessary. Moreover the lack of correlation of the *in vitro* with the *in vivo* data on products currently marketed does not give us hope that new products to come into commerce in the years ahead will necessarily give greater correlation than current dosage forms.

How far then must we go down this road of attempting to make correlations of *in vivo* and *in vitro* data? and how long must we wait till we find one that is satisfactory? At this time there is no answer to these questions, and it is an uncertain and clouded future.

One suggestion that has been made is that those who do bioavailability studies should keep large amounts of the dosage forms available, for release to those who claim to have predictive dissolution tests available. The viewpoint has some merit, and I am prepared to make available to some investigators samples of the dosage forms studied at the Food and Drug Directorate. Certain aspects of the question will always remain unanswered – did aging, storage, transportation, or any other factor have an effect on dissolution parameters measured at some point later in time?

Our research at FDD in Canada is devoted in the first phase to an evaluation of the bioavailability of currently marketed products of specially chosen drugs. Our most pressing long-term task is to attempt to define those circulating levels of drug which correlate with the fastest clinical improvement, and to recognize those physiological, biochemical, and genetic factors which could influence in one way or another such circulating levels to hinder clinical improvement or to cause toxic reactions.

References

1 *Oser, B.L.; Melnick, D., and Hochberg, M.:* Ind. Eng. Chem. *17:* 405 (1945).
2 *Lasagna:* Proc. Symp. Physiological Equivalence of Drug Dosage Forms, Ottawa 1969, Catalogue No. H44-2969 (Queen's Printer, and Controller of Stationary, Ottawa 1969).
3 R_X bulletin, January and February 1971 (Food and Drug Directorate, Department of National Health and Welfare, Ottawa 1971).
4 Second (final) report of the special committee of the House of Commons on drug costs and prices, p. 17 (Queen's Printer and Controller of Stationery, Ottawa 1967).
5 *Mattok, G.L.; McGilveray, I.J., and Charette, C.:* Clin. Chem. *16:* 822 (1970).
5a *Mattok, G.L.; Hossie, R.D., and McGilveray, I.J.:* Canad. J. pharm. Sci. (in press).
6 *Conklin, J.D. and Hollifield, R.D.:* Clin. Chem. *12:* 690 (1966).
7 *Wagner, J.G.:* Drug Intellig. *4:* 160 (1970).
8 *Petten, G.R. van; Feng, H.; Withey, R.J., and Lettau, H.F.:* J. clin. Pharmacol. *11:* 177 (1971).
8a *Withey, R.J.; Feng, H.; Cook, D.; Petten, G.R. van, and Lettau, H.F.:* J. clin. Pharmacol. *11:* 187 (1972).
9 *Mattok, G.L. and McGilveray, I.J.:* J. pharm. Sci. (in press).
10 *Mattok, G.L.; McGilveray, I.J., and Hossie, R.D.* (unpublished results).
11 *Mattok, G.L.; McGilveray, I.J., and Cook, D.:* Canad. J. pharm. Sci. *6:* 35 (1971).
12 *McGilveray, I.J.; Mattok, G.L.; Fooks, J.R.; Jordan, N., and Cook, D.:* Canad. J. pharm. Sci. *6:* 38 (1971).
13 *Mattok, G.L.; McGilveray, I.J., and Mainville, C.A.:* J. pharm. Sci. *60:* 561 (1971).

Author's address: Dr. *Denys Cook*, Chief, Pharmaceutical Chemistry Division, Food and Drug Directorate, Department of National Health and Welfare, *Tunney's Pasture, Ottawa 3, Ont.* (Canada)

Discussions

Question (audience): If we consider the case of a drug from a manufacturer where he is unable to obtain equal bioequivalence of two dosage forms, say a tablet and syrup, what would your advice be? If, for example, the syrup is only 70 % bioavailable relative to the tablet, should one equalize the two dosage forms by adding more active ingredient to the syrup? This perhaps could be accompanied by a label statement: Warning, contains 130 mg active ingredient, delivers 100 mg.

Response (Dr. Leeson): Something is wrong with the syrup dosage form and it behooves the company to find out what that is. Since the liquid is less bioavailable, this is obviously a problem which has to be overcome.

Comment (from panel): If for some reason you cannot solve the problem, perhaps one should decide which dose performs the therapeutic affect and this should be the (recognized or recommended) dose.

Question (audience): This is not the issue, this is a philosophical point. What should we do? State that the syrup delivers only 70 % or increase to 130 mg?

Response (Dr. Doluisio): But we are concerned with dose to the body, not dose on the label.

Question (audience): But is not the dose going to be determined by clinical trial regardless of whether or not you know the bioavailability of the dosage form?

Comment (panel): The problem may not be in the formulation. Since you have a liquid and are apparently obtaining less absorption, it may be that the transit time may be much shorter. It may be that the syrup should not even be on the market.

Comment (panel): The principle should be established that you have to state, that so much of the syrup is bioequivalent to one tablet. Perhaps someday we will have units of bioavailability rather than mg of active drug.

Question (audience): I wish to address this to Dr. *Cook.* Recently, in Canada, you published a listing of the drug quality assurance of various products with their prices and manufacturers. Have all the drug products for which you made such comparisons been rated for bioavailability by the FDD?

Response (Dr. Cook): No, the parameters measured were clearly stated in each issue. Most data were from analytical values. Few bioavailability studies can be done due to their cost and tediousness.

Question (audience): Perhaps you should change the label from drug quality assurance to something else.

Response (Dr. Cook): I knew we would have problems with the word assurance.

Question (audience): Ciba-Geigy deserves congratulations for making formulation changes [to phenylbutazone tablets, ed.] to improve their dosage form. Dr. *Leeson,* perhaps you could tell us about the concern a company experiences in making such changes.

Response (Dr. Leeson): A great deal of credit goes to the company (management) and to their willingness and the capability to go to the FDA to present new data.

Question (audience): This is addressed to Dr. *Conklin.* In your paper in 1969 you mentioned using a dosage schedule for nitrofurantoin of 1 tablet 4 times a day. Dr. *Cook* mentioned using a 100-mg tablet. Is there any advantage in using the 400-mg dose?

Response (Dr. Conklin): Are you referring to a comparison of bioavailability from a single dose to multiple dose?

Question (audience): No, Dr. *Cook*'s was a single dose and I believe yours was also.

Response (Dr. Conklin): No, ours was a multiple dose in order to evaluate urine drug excretion under simulated dosing conditions. At present, for simple urinary tract infections the drug is recommended for 7–10 days. As a result we administered the compound, 100 mg as tablet, for a 7-day period and checked urine on days 1 and 7.

Question (audience): Do you recommend this procedure?

Response (Dr. Conklin): In regard to bioavailability, with this drug it does not make much difference. Dr. *Cook* supports this. To the best of our knowledge the compound has a relatively short half-life even after it is administered for relatively long periods of time.

Question (audience): When a dosage formulation is changed as in the case of phenylbutazone, how much of a change is recommended in the dosage schedule?

Response (Dr. Leeson): No change, since there is no difference in bioavailability. The ultimate equilibrium blood level is the same; the drug just gets there more rapidly if the time between the doses is the same.

Comment (panel): Where the entire dose is not available, the clinical end of things has to be looked at very carefully in terms of a sharp alteration of dose schedule. This is a serious step that has to be considered.

Question (audience): You measured *in vitro* dissolution rates for nitrofurantoin, and *in vivo* levels based on urinary excretion. How about blood level data, was drug detectable and data reproducible?

Response (Dr. Cook): The trial was divided into three 7 × 7 Latin squares. Since urine distribution is easily measured it was used as the basis for the study. We have no figures for actual peak blood level but have figures for the time it takes to reach 30 μg/ml. Bioavailability data were compared using urinary excretion data and between 4 or 5 methods using different fluids.

Question (audience): Did you determine blood levels with tablets?

Response (Dr. Cook): I have no details. We plan to make data available in the literature in the form of surveys that are somewhat larger in scope than those you heard this morning.

Question (audience): Irrespective of the definition of bioavailability, it seems to me that we have to measure blood or urine levels. If a single dose gives us full bioavailability, is there any justification for multiple-dose experiments?

Response (panel): I can give a partial reply based on data presented yesterday. Under certain conditions, for the sake of simplicity, you may be faced with the need to do blood levels during a multiple-dose rather than single-dose schedule. This is in direct relationship to the half-life. For drugs with extremely long half-lives it is recommended that a few samples be taken during a multiple-dose schedule.

Comment (panel): There are many complexities in a multiple-dose study – you must get patients to the steady state and this takes about 5 half-lives. Furthermore, controls are more difficult.

Comment (panel): In the multiple-dose schedule, if you have a microsomal enzyme inhibitor, plasma levels may actually fall as you continue dosage. This needs to be known.

Comment (panel): To correlate between the two, the area between dosage intervals during a multiple-dose schedule should be equivalent to the area under single-dose curve, if we are dealing with a linear system.

Comment (panel): Unfortunately, variations in responses become greater during long dose periods.

Question (audience): This concerns the *in vitro* dissolution method. In view (to Dr. *Cook*) of your experience using 5 to 6 methods, is it likely that we will have a standard method and apparatus?

Response (Dr. Cook): The purpose of this meeting is to decide if out of the multiplicity of *in vitro* tests, we can focus on some that do give correlations with bioavailability – in this case, nitrofurantoin. There are two aspects to the dissolution test. If I have read USP correctly, in the case of this drug it says 'Thou shalt not dissolve more than a given amount in a given time'. In all other cases, it says you must dissolve at least a minimum amount which should be related to bioavailability. Furthermore, the monograph for nitrofurantoin still requires a disintegration test whereas the tendency is to remove this test from other monographs (where a dissolution requirement is given). Therefore, I am tempted to conclude that for nitrofurantoin the disintegration test is designed to guarantee bioavailability and the dissolution test to prevent reaching a high systemic or urine level too quickly due to side-effects. The second aspect is that all manufacturers should have a dissolution test but should we have one test or should the manufacturer decide on the test, apparatus, conditions and compliance to suit his needs?

Comment (Dr. Doluisio): It is interesting that all drugs discussed today are weak acids, and pH of dissolution medium of all dissolution tests was 7.4. However, I do not think any generalization can be drawn.

Comment (Dr. Leeson): I think that looking for a single dissolution rate test is foolish. You should develop one that correlates *in vivo* and *in vitro* data.

Question (audience): I have noted the emphasis on blood levels. However, there are a large number of drugs for which this has no correlation with pharmacologic effect, e.g. antibiotics, anticancer and antiviral agents. The active form may be a metabolite or a reaction product with some cellular constituent. What advice can you give for these categories of drugs?

Response (Dr. Leeson): This is a real and good point. L-dopa is another good example. You can have two preparations, one which is acted upon by decarboxylase in the stomach and is changed even before it is absorbed. Another preparation may pass through the stomach and then be absorbed rapidly. No firm conclusions can be made based on the presence of L-dopa in blood. One has to resort to therapeutic effect – this will be the basis for determining bioavailability of many products.

Comment (Dr. Doluisio): As more sensitive analytical techniques become available greater emphasis can be placed on correlating blood levels and therapeutic response.

Question (audience): A view which deserves to be considered stems from the pharmacologic approach. One should look at the clinical response of a drug with respect to dose as a dose-response type phenomenon. If one looks at bioavailability without respect to this point of view one neglects to observe those compounds with flat dose-response curves. But these are not really the subject of discussion here. One should worry about those with steep dose-response curves since 80–100 % can mean the difference between ineffective levels and side-effects.

Response (Dr. Doluisio): The point is well taken.

Dr. Weiner (from audience): I wish to make a comment and ask a question. It was no trouble at all to get Ciba-Geigy to change their formulation, it was merely a result of our free enterprise system. This way the competition will never have anything on you. I noticed, Dr. *O'Reilly*, that you administered dicumarol in a rapidly-absorbed formulation and also in a somewhat slower formulation. The peaks are at first day and $2^2/_3$ days. Since increase in absorption is only by a few hours, I find it hard to see how response is increased by a few days. I have done a lot of single dose i.v. dicumarol studies and do not remember a patient that responded maximally in less than 2 days.

Response (Dr. O'Reilly): I showed 3 curves, one each for solution, powder and tablet forms. Peak blood levels with tablets were 3–4 days. I believe you are alluding to peak levels with the powder – which is only a few hours different from the solution form. The peak effect goes deep into the clotting mechanism. We refer to a one-stage prothrombin time. There are at least four different vitamin K clotting factors. Ours is a reflection of factor 7. If you analyze degradation half-lives of clotting factors and assume that you shut off hepatic synthesis completely; in 24 h you can indeed reach prothrombin response above the 22-sec mark. In no way is it an anti-thrombotic effect which can be better correlated with (but not yet established) levels of prothrombin which take 5–6 days to fall off.

Comment (Dr. Wagner): I cannot agree with this. I do not believe one can mix bioavailability with pharmacologic response. Bioavailability relates to what is on the label in mg and to what gets to the body in mg – not response. You must divorce the two. Dose response and pharmacologic response are separate subjects and should be studied, but not confused with bioavailability.

Pharmacology 8: 199–214 (1972)

Panel Discussion on the Significance of Bioavailability

Moderator: *J.V. Bergen*, Washington, D.C. (USA)
Participants: *M. Weiner*, Ardsley, N.Y. (USA); *Thomas J. Macek*, Rockville, Md. (USA); *H.E. Simmons*, Rockville, Md. (USA); *C.A. Walton*, Lexington, Ky. (USA); *D.L. Azarnoff*, Kansas City, Kans. (USA)

Opening Remarks

J.V. Bergen
Section National Formulary, American Pharmaceutical Association, Washington, D.C.

We now move to a very important portion of the Conference on Bioavailability of Drugs: a panel discussion on the significance of bioavailability.

Before presenting very brief opening remarks and introducing the first of five panel members representing major segments of the pharmaceutical science and health care community, I would first like to use this opportunity to express publicly my personal and very grateful appreciation to the United States Pharmacopeia and the Drug Research Board – who have planned and organized this conference – for inviting me to serve as moderator of this final panel discussion which I consider an especially important part of the proceedings. Moreover, speaking on behalf of the National Formulary, we share with the other sponsors a vital interest in drug standards and in the significance of bioavailability, and welcome the opportunity to co-sponsor the conference program.

Along with its sister compendium – the USPh – the NF shares a 3-fold responsibility in assuring drug quality: (a) to the medical profession, so that it may have a high degree of confidence in the safety and effectiveness of drugs prescribed; (b) to the pharmacy profession, so that it may have confidence in the quality of drug products dispensed, and (c) most acutely to the public, whose health needs both professions exist to serve.

The NF is a project of the American Pharmaceutical Association and the entire profession of pharmacy, undertaken with the generous cooperation of the profession of medicine, the pharmaceutical industry, various governmental agencies including the food and drug administration, and the academic scientific community. It is through the NF revision program that APhA and the pharmacy profession seek to exercise their obligation in assuring to the maximum possible extent the quality of the drug supply to this nation. But the total scope of activities comprising the revision programs of the official compendia and other activities oriented toward achieving this objective constitutes a team effort, with the members of the team being those groups represented on the panel here this morning and on this entire conference program. More about this team effort in a moment.

The purpose of this conference is to focus on practical problems in producing specific drug products to meet uniform criteria of equivalent activity, and to explore guide lines for establishing requirements in the important area of drug bioavailability. Bioavailability generally involves other than the measure of clinical effects and the direct determination of therapeutic equivalence, an ideal but somewhat impractical goal for purposes of routine standardization. It involves other than chemical or physical tests which from the standpoint of routine standardization offer convenience, precision, and reproducibility. Rather it is something in between – a measure of drug product equivalence using blood levels or comparable measurements, as well as the real or potential possibility of correlation with clinical effects and chemical and physical parameters.

The inroads made by the discipline of biopharmaceutics in delineating and solving problems of bioavailability are great indeed. During the almost $1^1/_2$ days of this conference we have heard of some of these inroads from several of the most eminent scientists currently pursuing studies in the biopharmaceutics field. Indeed we have heard some intriguing suggestions; to name just two, the suggestion of Dr. *Levy* that a policy of full disclosure be adopted with regard to the status of bioavailability testing of individual drug articles, and the suggestion of Dr. *Barr* that reference standard dosage forms be made available for the purpose of characterizing and calibrating further dissolution studies and to enable control data on normal subjects to be obtained. Now, the question before us in this panel discussion is not *whether* bioavailability is significant but rather in *what manner* is it significant to the consumer as seen by the various members of the pharmaceutical science-health care team represented on the program. As noted by Dr. *Heller* in his welcoming remarks yesterday, an objective of this conference is to determine how the inroads of biopharmaceutics can be wedded to the practical needs of manufacturers, practitioners, and those agencies engaged in standards and enforcement activities so as to develop tests and standards which will optimize drug therapy.

In this connection we are going to hear from (a) Dr. *M. Weiner* representing the pharmaceutical industry, which must assume responsibility for demonstrating the safety and biological or clinical effectiveness of each marketed drug product; (b) Dr. *T.J. Macek* representing the official compendia which must assume responsibility for establishing public standards reflecting both the full capabilities of the industry and the most advanced scientific knowledge; (c) Dr. *H.E. Simmons* representing the food and drug administration to which the public has entrusted responsibility for judging the safety and efficacy claimed for each drug product; (d) Dr. *C.A. Walton* representing the profession of pharmacy which is assuming an increasing role in drug product selection and concomitantly finds an increasing need for bioavailability data pertaining to individual drug products, and (e) Dr. *D.L. Azarnoff* representing the profession of medicine to which the welfare of patients – including diagnosis, medical treatment, and drug therapy – is ultimately entrusted. These men represent most of the team segments to which I referred earlier; a team working together that has the public responsibility to ensure drug safety and efficacy, and to ensure to the maximum possible extent the therapeutic equivalence of comparable drug products.

In opening this panel discussion, a very recent editorial (1) entitled 'Comparability and consensus' is pertinent. It said in part: 'Medicine shows two faces to the world – the scientific (discovery) and the technological (practice) – interdependent activities that demand compatibility if each is to endure and grow. Science builds on hypothesis, study, validation. Practice requires art – the wisdom to apply knowledge to an individual, a group, or a community so as to achieve optimum results.'

The editorial went on to conclude: 'If ever there were a need for consensus on behalf of medicine, it is now. Without consensus, we face the evils of inconsistent goals and a likelihood of inner incompatibilities.'

Avoiding these 'inner incompatibilities' is what the panel discussion today is all about!

Reference

1 *Anon:* J. amer. med. Ass. *218:* 1044 (1971).

Author's address: Dr. *John V. Bergen*, Director, National Formulary, 2215 Constitution Avenue, N.W., *Washington, DC 20037* (USA)

Pharmaceutical Industry

M. Weiner
Department of Biologic Research, Geigy Pharmaceuticals, Ciba-Geigy Corporation, Ardsley, N.Y.

In the late 1940s I had the good fortune to train as a hemotologist at Goldwater Memorial Hospital where there was a great deal of interest in the biochemical approach to problems of drug therapy. I was intrigued by the fact that the clotting response to a single oral dose of dicumarol could not be detected for ten or more hours; it generally took several days to reach its peak, and the effect lasted for days afterwards. I was delighted when *Julius Axelrod*, working in Dr. *B.B. Brodie*'s laboratory at the hospital, called me to say he had developed a fairly simple u.v. absorption method for estimating the concentration of dicumarol in plasma. Our subsequent studies of intravenous versus oral blood levels (1, 2) indicated that the drug was generally but not invariably completely absorbed, had a rather long half-life, and showed considerable individual patient variations in blood levels achieved. Blood levels peaked before any clotting response was apparent and the clotting responses lasted for 1–2 days after the drug was no longer detectable in the blood. While a correlation could be made between the duration of the clotting response and the persistence of measurable blood levels, it was not possible to predict the intensity of the clotting response from the blood levels from subject to subject, and several apparent conflicts with existing theory of drug disposition were noted. For example, the half-life of the drug varied with dose in the same individuals and this difference was reflected in the fact that with continuous daily dosage, doubling the dose led to more than double the so-called plateau plasma level. Subsequent studies (3) with another long half-life drug, phenylbutazone, showed the reverse phenomenon, i.e. doubling the dose led to much less than double the plasma levels, in spite of which, larger doses are more toxic. We also showed quite clearly that the clotting effect with the coumarin-type anticoagulants can be cumulative even when plasma levels of the drug are not cumulative (4). These variables exemplify the complexity of factors which must be considered in planning and interpreting bioavailability studies.

The many subsequent studies with these drugs were indeed fascinating and threw considerable light on the mechanisms of drug action. But, in the last analysis, the control of anticoagulant dosage remains now as it was then, a question of following the appropriate physiological parameter, i.e. clotting tests, and not the drug blood levels in each individual.

From the point of view of the drug producer, however, bioavailability evaluations by blood level determinations have become very important. When the anticoagulant phenylindandione was first manufactured and tested in the US, initial observations suggested that approximately half the patients were resistant to the drug as prepared. Our bioavailability studies with this drug in the early 1950s (5) clearly demonstrated that the tablet used, which passed the usual disintegration standards of that time, was inconsistently and incompletely absorbed in contrast to other preparations of the active ingredient studied in crossover in man. There was no question after the study of this tablet in single doses in 3 or 4 patients, that erratic clinical results could be expected on the basis of poor bioavailability. While many more patients and experimental points are needed to derive the constants for the equation of Dr. *Wagner* it took only four to prove the formulation was no good. In an area such as anticoagulant therapy, where there are tremendous biologic variations influencing individual response to the drug, it is very easy for inadequacies in bioavailability to be submerged and escape clinical detection. This fact does not excuse the further confounding of the variables which are beyond the control of the clinician by giving him less than reliably absorbed formulations. I think the drug producer has a very real responsibility to define and control to the greatest degree he can, *within practical limits,* the properties of his products so that the physician will have one less variable to worry about in his difficult task of using drugs in a heterogeneous population.

In seeking this goal, the producer must use all his ingenuity in designing *in vivo* and *in vitro* tests which will best fit the particular clinical utility for which each medication is intended, taking into account the nature of the chemical. A very important step in accomplishing this purpose is to develop knowledge wherever possible, of the bioavailability patterns which the drug can yield and the therapeutic implications which *may* make one pattern more desirable than the other for a particular purpose with the particular drug. In his enthusiasm to develop and apply this information, the scientists must not lose sight of the very real limits to what can be accomplished with bioavailability. Limits are imposed by the state of the relevant analytic art and the disposition characteristics of the particular drug which must be considered in the interpretation of blood levels and urinary excretion patterns of the drug and its metabolites as reflections of bioavailability.

For each drug two important questions should be asked: (1) what pattern of absorption is therapeutically desirable, and (2) how can it be achieved. In general, the more rapidly a drug is absorbed, the more rapidly will the therapeutic effect commence. Complete absorption is obviously desirable in order to achieve true dose control. The longer absorption is delayed, the more likely that some fraction of the dose will be unabsorbed in some patients. With short-acting drugs, it is occasionally desirable to prolong absorption in order to obtain a smoother continuing response and to eliminate the tops of short-lived but excessive levels which may be associated with side-effects. However, when drug half-life is long, compared to dose interval, there is rarely any advantage in delayed absorption. With preparations which may be locally irritating to the gastrointestinal tract, a longer 'residence time' in the gut before absorption may mean increased opportunity for local irritation.

While these considerations can be helpful in determining the most desired bioavailability pattern, one must remember that even with the same drug the pattern most desirable for one set of circumstances may be different for another. Rapid disintegration and dissolution can be a critical advantage up to a point, a possible advantage beyond that point, and of no further advantage or even a disadvantage if carried still further. A tablet which disintegrates in seconds can be a handicap to those few people whose skill in swallowing tablets is not adequate to prevent a distasteful disintegration in the mouth and throat before it is swallowed. I know of instances where this complaint has led to a selection of one brand of aspirin over another by some patients, and the opposite selection by other patients who found the more rapidly disintegrating and dissoluting brand less of a gastric irritant. One of these brands should not be classified as 'better' than the other. A regulatory demand that all brands be reliably absorbed is reasonable. A demand that they have *identical* characteristics is neither wise nor just. Bioavailability studies, *per se,* cannot solve the artificial problem of determining a 'best' product and demanding that all preparations be identical to it.

There are examples where two different formulations studied in the same group of patients yielded essentially the same average results, but with a distinct, statistically significantly greater degree of individual variations around the means with one formulation as compared to the other. While one could argue that it might be very difficult to demonstrate clinical differences in efficacy between two such formulations, I am sure any physician would prefer having the formulation which is more consistent in its pattern of absorption. Certainly, no one denies the fact that a 100 mg tablet produced with a range limit of 95–105 mg is a preferred product to one which can be produced more cheaply with a range limit of 70–130 mg, even though in many instances it would be difficult to demonstrate a statistically significant difference in clinical efficacy between these tablets. Of course, this concept can be carried to a 'zero tolerance' hairsplitting and hair-raising extreme in the other direction. A formulation with a less reliable bioavailability pattern may be therapeutically satisfactory, but should not be accepted as completely equivalent simply because therapeutic non-equivalence had not yet been demonstrated.

Biochemical bioavailability studies in a few subjects can be most reassuring in determining the equivalence of two similar but not identical formulations or materials prepared under significantly different conditions. A new formulation should be demonstrably equivalent to an older one by some appropriate test before it is accepted as equivalent. By and large, the demonstration that blood level patterns are essentially the same, can be taken as evidence that bioavailability is the same, even if the design and numbers are not adequate for calculation of a variety of sophisticated theoretical mathematical constants. Since there are differences in the state of analytic art, patterns of drug disposition, and mechanisms of action from compound to compound, biochemical bioavailability studies should not be an automatic regulatory requirement for all drugs. Objection to legal regulations which will have the effect of a fixed blind demand for specific studies is not only consistent with a high respect for the value of bioavailability studies, but is essential to avoid the misapplication of such studies to inappropriate situations.

It is the history of almost every new scientific approach that it is first greeted with skepticism by those who do not understand it, followed by over-enthusiasm as a flicker of light dawns and the bandwagon comes into sight. Then there is a period of disappointment when the rough edges become visible, followed finally by an understanding of the true value and limitations of the new tool. Considering the present state of the art, the development of standards to help in the design and interpretation of bioavailability studies can best take the form of cataloging the lessons learned to date with a variety of well-studied compounds. The need for detailed cookbook bioavailability guide lines is directly proportional to the incompetence of the investigator or the reviewer. Whether a method and design of study is good or bad can only be evaluated in the light of the questions it purports to answer, and these questions differ markedly with the drug and the particular problem.

The time has come for a reasoned dispassionate acceptance of what bioavailability has to offer. It can and already has led to major improvements in the drugs available to the American people. It can also lead to a waste of untold thousands of precious scientific man-hours, if studies are done to fulfill misguided fixed requirements rather than to answer important specific scientific questions.

We are at the crossroads. I hope we will have the wisdom and the courage to go the right way.

References

1 *Weiner, M.; Shapiro, S.; Axelrod, J.; Cooper, J., and Brodie, B.:* The physiological disposition of dicumarol in man. J. Pharmacol. exp. Ther. *99:* 409 (1950).

2 *Weiner, J.; Brodie, B.B., and Burns, J.J.:* A comparative study of hypoprothrombinemic agents. Proc. 1st Int. Congr. Thrombosis and Embolism, Basle 1954, p. 181.

3 *Brodie, B.; Lowman, E.; Burns, J.; Lee, P.; Chenkin, T.; Coldman, A.; Weiner, M., and Steele, J.:* Observations on the antirheumatic and physiologic effects of phenylbutazone (butazolidin) and some comparisons with cortisone. Amer. J. Med. *16:* 181 (1954).

4 *Brodie, B.; Weiner, M.; Burns, J.; Simpson, G., and Yale, E.:* The physiological disposition of ethyl biscoumacetate (tromexan) in man and a method for its estimation in biological material. J. Pharmacol. exp. Ther. *106:* 453 (1952).

5 *Schulert, A. and Weiner, M.:* The physiologic disposition of phenylindanedione in man. J. Pharmacol. exp. Ther. *110:* 451 (1954).

Author's address: Dr. *Murray Weiner,* Vice President, Merrell-National Laboratories, *Cincinnatti, OH 45215* (USA)

The Official Compendia

T.J. Macek
The United States Pharmacopeia, Rockville, Md.

The spotlight of public attention no longer shines brightly upon the miracle drugs and the great drug discoveries of our times. If focuses instead on drug formulations and on product equivalence. There is today a realization and the mundane acknowledgment that drugs are seldom, if ever, administered to man except as formulations. It is conceded that the different binders and excipients that surround the active ingredient and the manner in which drug products are formulated can significantly influence how that active ingredient is absorbed in the body.

When the new drug requirements were first introduced into the Food and Drug Act in 1938 there was established a new emphasis and priority on drug safety. Nevertheless, if one firm marketed a drug product which, by experience, was recognized as safe, then similar preparations produced by other firms with the same drug substance and identified by the same common name, were also usually regarded as safe. Many duplicate products soon appeared. For example, the reserpine tablet products number more than 50, and there are more than 45 meprobamate tablet products currently on the domestic market. After all, these products had the same common name and conformed to the same compendial specifications. Their compositions, from what, and how they had been made, and their bioavailability, had not been, and did not become, a critical point at issue. The emphasis on formulation factors and bioavailability was coincident largely with the new drug amendments that later, in addition to safety, focused attention on the proof of efficacy. The controversy over product equivalence resulted from this and from many other complex considerations, including economic factors.

The challenge now facing us is simply this. When drug products are not equivalent, in the best interest of the patient, what must be done to assure their optimal equivalence?

Several decades ago an awareness and recognition of the problem, and the subsequent development and acceptance of good public standards, served to wipe out the then widespread occurrence of drug adulteration. We seldom hear of problems of outright drug adulteration any more. Similarly, what appears to be needed now are standards for bioavailability in order to assure drug product uniformity and equivalence. The question is how can this best be accomplished, and how can the compendia, as standards-setting organizations representing the professions, best serve the interests of the public as well in this urgent and important task? From my standpoint, there is no other, single, more important matter facing the compendia today than the development of objective standards by means of which the bioavailability of drug products, where there is a problem, can be measured and expressed in clear and unmistakable language.

The need for such standards was recognized by the compendia during the previous revision period. Accordingly, a USP/NF joint panel on physiological availability was appointed and tried vainly to make progress. Unfortunately, the work of this panel did not succeed in producing standards for *in vivo* testing as had been hoped for, but resulted instead in dissolution tests and requirements for 13 official formulations. Perhaps there was a lack of a full understanding of the problem and the possible solutions by all concerned. Some, no doubt, will say that we are still too premature in attempting to develop standards even now. Nevertheless, I believe that we have a new opportunity in this new revision period for a new start, to consider again the development of bioavailability requirements. This can be done by means of a cooperative process involving the compendia where all voices are heard, leading to the definition of meaningful public tests and standards for the benefit of all concerned.

The dissolution requirements of the USP and NF have been criticized as being of little consequence. Correlations with bioavailability are implied, it is claimed, without adequate justification. Indeed, the USP even states that since drug absorption and physiological availability are largely dependent upon having the drug in the dissolved state, suitable dissolution characteristics are an important property of a satisfactory drug product.

In some instances the criticism may be justified, but it is equally certain that dissolution testing has been misapplied and misrepresented by numerous investigators as well as producers. It has been used far beyond its means, and the time has come for corrective action.

The bioavailability of a drug product can only be assessed by biological testing, and preferably in man. This is the primary requirement. If we are fortunate and should find or develop *in vitro* tests, dissolution or otherwise, that can be shown to correlate with the *in vivo* findings, then such physical tests will be extremely useful for measuring the batch-to-batch uniformity of product in a way that has unusual significance. Anything other than that is merely a physical test for drug release, and perhaps should even be called that instead of dissolution. In order to have meaningful *in vitro* tests and requirements, the biological tests must be achieved first.

The many difficult problems associated with the testing of bioavailability and the comparative equivalence of two or more products of the same drug in man have been documented adequately by numerous authors. It has been concluded that it is unrealistic to consider, and impossible to conduct, tests in humans on every batch of even the troublesome products. If tests in humans constitute the only reliable means of demonstrating equivalence, so we are told, an unacceptably large burden will be imposed upon the drug manufacturers and the clinical-testing facilities. But it also follows that until the time when there become available suitable, well-defined testing methods and protocols, in order to evaluate different formulations of the same drug substance in man, it is unlikely that we shall be in a position to objectively assess non-equivalence between products, and accordingly the uncertainties and discourse will continue.

I believe that the time has come for the description of standard reference methods for testing the bioavailability of specific drugs in the compendia. These should be complete in every respect, detailing design of the clinical test, the numbers and kinds of patients, their physiological state, the drug-dosage regimen, sampling procedures and intervals, analytical methods in detail, and calculations and interpretation of the data and findings. The use of a reference preparation of the drug substance itself, in this kind of a test, will serve to equate the unknown product to an acceptable reference, just as in any other, well-defined, and recognized compendial assay. Comparative bioavailability testing against a given commercial 'standard product', even though FDA-approved as safe and effective, assumes that the standard product is sufficiently well-controlled from the standpoint of bioavailability in its batch-to-batch and dose-to-dose variations so that it is fully reproducible. This, I think, is assuming too much; the quality of the reference standard must be known with certainty, and must be unequivocal. Indeed, certain commercial drug products have gained a wide degree of acceptance even though they may not exist in the optimum dosage form or be administered in a dosage regimen that is ideal for maximal clinical effect.

When developed, the standard reference bioavailability tests should be used sparingly. A new producer entering the market would be required to provide data to show that his product qualifies to bear the common name, and is equivalent and available. The method would be employed, perhaps, in support of a significant change in product composition or in the process of manufacture. There should be few doubts about this since it is already being done by the conscientious manufacturer. The method would serve in a referee capacity whenever there is a valid question of differences in product identity or quality. The method would serve as a common denominator for demonstrating product equivalence. In fact, on the basis of such analysis, as our thinking and testing become more refined, we may discover that what is now identified as non-equivalence in some cases may result in the identification and definition of distinct and different products of a common drug entity. This now would become a matter of accurate and meaningful drug product identification and labeling.

The compendia seek the cooperation of all concerned in this difficult but essential endeavor, but stand ready to move ahead in our unique enterprise of establishing privately the standards for drugs that are then recognized and enforced under the law.

Author's address: Dr. *Thomas J. Macek,* Director of Revision, The United States Pharmacopeia, 12601 Twinbrook Parkway, *Rockville, MD 20852* (USA)

Food and Drug Administration

H.E. Simmons

Food and Drug Administration, Bureau of Drugs, Rockville, Md.

It is a pleasure for me to have the opportunity to discuss with you some aspects of bioavailability and also to describe some of the goals of the FDA in this area.

At its annual meeting in 1968, the APS of the APhA adopted the following policy statement: 'Prior to the initial distribution of a drug product, or modifications of an existing product, every manufacturer should be obligated to perform tests which are appropriate and sufficient to demonstrate the clinical safety and efficacy claimed for that manufacturer's product. In particular, in the absence of such tests, it cannot be assumed that the product will exhibit clinical acceptability simply because an apparently identical product is already marketed.'

We at the FDA are in basic agreement with that statement. The time has long since passed when chemical equivalence can provide assurance of therapeutic equivalence. You are all aware of examples of chemical equivalence of marketed drugs which fail to yield biological equivalence and have heard of many such instances discussed at this meeting. You are also aware of the multiplicity of factors which can influence bioavailability, and I shall not take the time to reiterate them here.

Bioavailability has come into its own as a reliable and legitimate method of drug testing and has been demonstrated to be an indispensable and scientifically-sound approach to assuring the biological or therapeutic equivalence of chemically identical drug products. It is here to stay. Continued experience with deficient products among established drug classes underscores the need for bioavailability. We depend on it to assure ourselves that chemically identical drug products are equally effective clinically. Bioavailability helps give us this assurance and does it expeditiously and economically. We feel that bioavailability testing will be a viable alternative to the need for periodic retesting of drugs and to clinical trials.

I believe that bioavailability has not received proper recognition as one of the most significant recent advances in drug research and development. Drug originators have found it indispensable to evaluate different dosage forms, to determine an effective dosage regimen, to confirm continued quality of modified drug formulations and to guard against reduction of quality of drug products during their shelf life. For these many reasons we, at the FDA also consider it important.

We realize that there are many questions yet to be answered in this area. We plan to help develop some of those answers, and the new information generated will certainly affect bioavailability policies which we will develop. Our new requirements of bioavailability may tax the talent available in this country to plan and do well the necessary studies. We are already working with a number of experts in this country to help us develop adequate methodology and to test the important drugs in question. We are counseling widely, and I think wisely, in this area, so that the policy on which we finally settle is scientifically sound. We hope to help develop some standard methodology in this area which can be made available to all. We see an obligation to avoid as much as possible any waste of valuable scientific resources.

We feel that definite benefits will accrue to the public and the profession as new bioavailability requirements are introduced. The physician and his patient will be more assured that the drugs prescribed in this country will behave in a more predictable fashion. In this rapidly changing and expanding field I see at least two absolutes at the present time: firstly, the more we look for problems in this area, the more we find, and secondly, the present policies of the FDA will, and indeed must, change to reflect that new knowledge.

Over the past few years there have been a wide variety of proposals as to what kind of bioavailability policy should be adopted. The various recommendations cover a wide range of possibilities. One group advocates that every batch of every drug of every manufacturer should undergo bioavailability testing, while others go to the opposite extreme and say it really does not make that much sense, it is not that important, let us go with the chemical equivalence alone. Somewhere between these two poles there must be a sensible workable policy. We at the FDA plan to do the best we can to develop a policy which would give the biggest yield, given the limitations of the field, and the resources at hand. The discussions of this conference will be helpful to us in defining such a policy.

Author's address: Dr. *Henry E. Simmons,* FDA, Bureau of Drugs, 5600 Fishers Lane, *Rockville, MD 20852* (USA)

The Profession of Pharmacy

Charles A. Walton, Ph.D.
University of Kentucky Medical Center, Lexington, Ky.

During the early years of my teaching career I spent quite a few summers in community and hospital pharmacies. In more recent years it has been possible for me to remain in contact with the technical and professional concerns of the pharmacy practitioner through my students (who are dedicated to keeping my courses relevant) and as a result of my participation in the work of our drug information center. This service supports our own hospital professionals and provides toll-free, direct-dial access to these services for health care practitioners throughout the Commonwealth of Kentucky. I believe it is possible for me to relate reasonably well some of the practitioner's views on the significance of bioavailability as it bears upon the profession of pharmacy. From some of the comments coming from this podium and dropped in the corridors during the past 2 days it appears that many persons are unaware of the sophisticated level of service which is currently provided by some of our younger pharmacists, particularly those who hold the Doctor of Pharmacy degree. It is also possible that some of our friends in the scientific disciplines outside of pharmacy are not too familiar with the progress that has been made in biopharmaceutics and pharmacokinetics in the last decade. Hopefully the opportunities afforded by this conference to review the subjects will remedy some of these communication deficits.

It is tempting to use this forum as a means of focusing attention on the young innovators in pharmacy practice and their desperate needs for more biopharmaceutical information and product performance data. I am, for example, much impressed by the reduction in medication errors in Ohio State's unit dose/medication administration program, the growing sophistication of drug information services in California, the improved quality of services in clinical practice in North Carolina and Buffalo, and new out-reach patient-care projects in many areas. Optimization of patient care with drugs could be materially improved in these and other aspects of newer pharmacy services were we able to provide them with better product information.

Because time does not permit me to discuss even the more important implications of bioavailability in these evolving concepts of professional pharmacy services I have chosen to limit my remarks to the frustrating predicament of the typical practitioner who must resort to empiricism in product selection because of the paucity of data supportive of rational approaches to this service requirement.

Pharmacists will readily acknowledge an essentially total lack of bioavailability data sufficient to characterize the relative therapeutic capabilities of the products which they distribute on prescription and otherwise. Although modern education and training convince them that currently available information on products is inadequate for rational assessment of alternative products, they are nonetheless, compelled to choose and dispense drugs as a major part of their role in society, and this they accomplish in a totally empirical manner. Objectively scrutinized, the product selection process appears to rest ultimately on four assumptions: (a) in the absence of specific data on bioavailability one must assume confidence in the knowledge, skills and reliability of well-established (usually larger) manufacturers; (b) the official compendia can be relied upon to include the essential, clinically relevant criteria as standards of dosage-form performance; (c) the practicalities of economics are necessary considerations in determining the quality of patient-care with drug products, and (d) accumulated clinical experiences constitute valid evidence of efficacy in the absence of specific product performance data.

These are almost precisely the circumstances which, over the years, have tended to shape the character of drug-prescribing practices and have led to the removal from the market of a number of popular remedies, which precipitated considerable criticism of the medical profession, and prompted *Dowling* (1) to conclude that '... a substantial proportion of doctors practice poor therapeutics by any reasonable standard'.

I find it reasonable to conclude that pharmacists practice poor biopharmaceutics by any reasonable standard.

Through many years of close association which hundreds of pharmacists of variable academic qualifications, ages, orientation to commercial aspects of their occupation, and intensity of altruistic commitment, I can truthfully state that I have never met one who, in my opinion, would knowingly dispense an ineffective product. It is my honest feeling that pharmacists abide by their professional code of ethics in its assertion that 'a pharmacist should never condone the dispensing, promoting or distributing of drugs or medical devices, or assist therein, which are not of good quality, which do not meet standards required by law or which lack therapeutic value for the patient' (2). The product selection problem as I see it is not one of professional negligence; rather it is one of inadequate scientific information on the basis of which intelligent professional judgments could be made.

In the absence of scientific evidence to the contrary, confidence in the products of well-established manufacturers does not seem irrational to me. The probabilities of procuring a quality product appear greater where the operation includes these three elements: (a) product design and development; (b) a production and in-process control, and (c) finished product testing. These three prerequisites for marketing a quality product are emphasized in the publication 'Drug Product Quality', prepared by the Academy of Pharmaceutical Sciences and endorsed by the American Pharmaceutical Association's House of Delegates (3). The fact that confidence in manufacturers whose operations provide for these three functions may not always be substantiated in practice is a matter of common knowledge and regularly repeated confirmation. Nonetheless, one sees evidence that most pharmacists continue to hold to this empirical basis for product selection in spite of its inherent inadequacies.

Reliance on the limited clinical relevance of compendia specifications is another source of error in attempting product selection. The inadequacies of such data not only limit professional judgment, they also tend to obscure the problem by appearing to provide reassurance in assessment of products. Although ascribing certain standards of quality to USP preparations, most pharmacists largely ignore the official compendia as sources of assistance in selecting products. I personally became acutely aware of such limitations many years ago as a student in pharmacy and in ROTC. To accomplish the purpose of a 155 mm artillery round I soon came to understand the importance of the projectile construction, weight, temperature, fuzing and shape. And although it was obviously important to control disintegration characteristics, it was obvious that none of these considerations of internal ballistics made much difference if the delivery system, the weapon, and external influences were excluded from computations. In trying to draw analogies between my artillery lessons and my pharmacy studies there seemed to be some valid comparisons; the delivery system is as essential as the active component. Even in the biopharmaceutically unsophisticated days of the late 1940s I found it difficult to accept the incredible compounding schemes designed to keep two or more obviously hostile physicochemical entities sufficiently dispersed to permit periodic ejection into a teaspoon. With the enlightenment provided in recent years by bioavailability research it is increasingly difficult to accept the assumptions of extemporaneous compounding or understand the continued absence from official compendia of relevant bioavailability data which could challenge some of these assumptions. As more and more data of this kind are generated and incorporated in the compendia, pharmacists will begin to return to these references as practical guides in professional practice.

The third element of empirical product selection relates to practicalities of economics. Depending upon state laws, budgets and the regulations of various third-party payees, alternatives in the selection of products will vary from one region to another. The pressure on reducing drug costs has been intensified by the concentration of purchasing responsibility, and it is unlikely that the pattern will change in the foreseeable future. As the final common pathway of drug distribution, the practicing pharmacist finds himself caught between diminishing reimbursement schedules and the responsibility of dispensing an expensive product of assumed quality rather than a chemical equivalent in which he has less confidence. In the absence of unequivocal comparative evidence he can be convincing in his contention that the less expensive product probably permits the most good to be done for the greatest number of patients in the system.

Just as he has stuck intuitively to confidence in major manufacturers in spite of occasional product recalls (4), he appears to be equally resolute in assuming performance equivalency of chemically identical entities where only a handful of exceptions have been conclusively proven.

Exemplifying this aspect of empiricism in drug product selection is a memorandum (5) issued to Ohio physicians and pharmacists on 8 November 1971, by the Director, Ohio Department of Public Welfare. The communication includes the following statement:

> We believe that economies can be achieved in the drug program if the professions *will prescribe and dispense by generic name* those drugs which consistently demonstrate therapeutic effectiveness and are produced by pharmaceutical manufacturers with strict quality controls. In filling such generic prescriptions the pharmacist is expected to dispense the least expensive generic drug available in his stock.

In the succeeding paragraph of this memorandum are listed 18 drugs which are 'examples of some of the most frequently prescribed and dispensed generic drugs'. Included are the following 10 drugs: digitoxin, digoxin, prednisolone, prednisone, reserpine, rauwolfia serpentina, sulfisoxazole, tetracycline, chloral hydrate and meprobamate.

This listing was of special interest because I had just recently had the opportunity to review a draft of 'Considerations in Drug Product Selection by Pharmacists' (6), a slide presentation under preparation by the Committee on Drug Product Equivalence of the APhA Academy of Pharmaceutical Sciences. In the text of this paper, the authors present examples of drug products with established 'potential for significant therapeutic differences'. If I understand this discipline at all, the authors of this document are trying to tell us that good quality controls would not necessarily prevent significant clinical differences among these products. It is interesting to note that the first 4 drugs in the Ohio list are included among the 8 drugs considered by the APS authors as possessing a 'high potential for significant therapeutic differences'. And as we all know, digitalis glycosides and corticosteroids are far from innocuous drugs. Another 4 drugs in the Ohio list are considered to have a 'moderate potential for therapeutic differences', and 2 are considered to have a low potential (but still capable of significant performance differences).

Now it may be legitimately argued that it is the physician rather than the pharmacist who must be responsible for the clinical performance of the products he prescribes. For a growing segment of our society it is obvious from the preceding discussion and an abundance of evidence elsewhere that such is in fact not the case. Moreover, it would appear to me that the pharmacist has been making these decisions for many years before Medicare, Medicaid and other such programs were inaugurated.

In 1964, *Hrebenach and Kenna* (7) reported a survey of drug distribution in the University of Chicago hospitals and clinics in which their orders were categorized by proprietary versus nonproprietary prescribing.

Of approximately 180 products stocked in their pharmacy which *could* have been purchased on a bid basis, 144 actually *were procured* by this method. They determined that

9 of these 144 were usually ordered by proprietary name (group A); 14 were ordered by proprietary name about 50 % of the time (group B), and 121 were usually ordered by nonproprietary name (group C). They estimated, on the basis of purchase records, that 93.1 % of all doses (a count of over 4.6 million), among products obtained on a bid basis and distributed in their service during the survey period, could be accounted for among the group C drugs, i.e. those which were usually prescribed by generic name.

Among the list of group C drugs I found seven of the eight drugs which the authors of the paper (6) on problems of drug product equivalence classified as having a 'high potential for significant therapeutic differences'. The eighth was listed in the Chicago survey among those drugs prescribed by proprietary name approximately 50 % of the time.

My final comment on empirical selection of products relates to the treachery of clinical impression as the basis for product acceptance. I could express it no better than *Lasagna* (8) who says, 'Scientific truth is not arrived at by a majority vote. There is too much evidence that the medical profession, like the rest of us, can be misled by "practical experience" to encourage the testing of truth by referendum. Our "experience" tells us that the earth is flat and that we are not spinning around in space, but neither of these happens to be true.'

References

1 *Dowling, H.F.:* How doctors use drugs: a perspective. Proc. Conference on Continuing Education for Physicians in the Use of Drugs, Washington, D.C. 1969.
2 Code of Ethics, American Pharmaceutical Association; in *Myers* Ethics; in *Gibson* Remington's pharmaceutical sciences; 14th ed., p. 23 (Mack, Easton 1970).
3 Anonym: Drug product quality. J. amer. pharm. Ass. *10:* 107 (1970).
4 *Chisholm, J.S.:* Quality control and drug recalls. Hosp. Form. Manage. *3:* 25 (1968).
5 *Hansan, J.E.:* Memorandum to Ohio Physicians and Pharmacists, Columbus 1971.
6 *Doluisio, J.T.:* Considerations in drug product selection by pharmacists (personal communication).
7 *Hrebenach, D.B. and Kenna, F.R.:* A study on brand specification and the hospital formulary system. Amer. J. Hosp. Pharmacy *21:* 163 (1964).
8 *Lasagna, L.:* Problems of drug development. Science *145:* 362 (1964).

Author's address: Dr. *Charles A. Walton,* Department of Oral Biology, College of Dentistry, University of Kentucky Medical Center, *Lexington, KY 40506* (USA)

The Profession of Medicine

D.L. Azarnoff
University of Kansas Medical Center, Kansas City, Kans.

The goal of the physician in treating any patient is firstly to make the correct diagnosis and secondly to select and administer the right drug in the right dosage and form at the right intervals. He expects the product to be therapeutically equivalent each time it is administered to the same patient. In selecting a drug, the physician wishes his patient to receive a high quality product at the lowest reasonable cost. By high quality he means the product he has selected should: (1) contain the active drug as well as any other component substances in the highest grade of purity; (2) contain the stated amount of active drug, and (3) be formulated so that the active component is readily and reproducibly available. Thus, he expects to be reasonably sure that any variation in pharmacological response is due to interpatient variability rather than intertablet, suspension or capsule variability. The number of drug product recalls by the FDA makes it quite evident that errors occur not infrequently in at least the first two categories and probably in the third, although systematic checks on this category are not done.

Is it enough to be reasonably certain that the amount of biologically available drug in any one product is reproducible? The physician is awakening to knowledge that biopharmaceutical formulations can greatly change the bioavailability of a drug product to the point where a drug ordered by prescription may have no effect, the desired therapeutic effect, or even a toxic effect depending upon which formulation of the drug is dispensed. At the same time, he is being cajoled and even coerced to prescribe by generic name. Although I firmly believe physicians should always prescribe by generic name, they should also indicate the manufacturer of the product they wish dispensed. If he prescribes by generic name alone, the physician cannot be sure at the present time that a patient going to one pharmacy will receive a product therapeutically equivalent to a patient going to a different pharmacy or even that the same patient will receive a therapeutically equivalent product each time he has his prescription filled at the same pharmacy. All too often I have seen well-controlled patients on a specific drug for months or years suddenly develop toxicity. Obviously, drug interactions and many other factors could account for the change, but the possibility of a recent change in the drug product the patient is receiving is always high on my list of suspected etiologies.

Today, as more and more chronic illnesses are being treated prophylactically as well as therapeutically with chronic, long-term drug therapy, the physician is becoming increasingly aware of drug product variability and the need for uniform standards. If meaningful standards are developed, he could then be satisfied that when he prescribed the right dosage form for the right disorder, the drug would be present not only in the correct amount and purity, but also be reproducibly available for absorption. Even though with our present knowledge we can only assume that a drug with equivalent bioavailability has therapeutic equivalency, it would be a significant step toward improving therapy. To develop the best standards it will be necessary, in some instances, to require changes in preparations physicians have used for many years. The rationale for such changes must be carefully documented if the physician is to accept them readily.

I would be remiss in my obligation to the patient if I did not at least mention in a conference on bioavailability that an elegant biopharmaceutic preparation is not the end of the line. That preparation must still be gotten into the patient and it is well known that patient compliance to dosage schedules is poor, even if they do take the medication. Other problems also exist. How many of you have ever tried to administer 0.025 mg digoxin to a 2-day-old infant? In one preparation, that dose is given in 0.5 ml. With a drug such as digoxin where the therapeutic-toxicity ratio is quite low, a dropper with calibrations can lead to significant error in a 0.5-ml dose. A simple expedient as diluting the drug so the same amount is in 1 ml would reduce the error one half.

In conclusion, meaningful bioavailability standards will improve and, in the long-run, reduce the cost of patient care by making it more likely for a patient to get the right amount of medicine, no matter whose preparation he receives, since an inadequate, as well as too great an amount, may prolong his illness. Physicians can only applaud efforts directed at preparing meaningful bioavailability standards.

Author's address: Dr. *Daniel L. Azarnoff*, Department of Medicine and Pharmacology, University of Kansas Medical Center, 39th and Rainbow Boulevard, *Kansas City, KS 66103* (USA)

Discussion

Comment (Dr. Gilman, from audience): Consumer protection agencies that support legislation for obligatory generic prescribing – denying physicians the knowledge of the source of the generic drug – have no concept of the risk/benefit ratio. At present such an attitude is dangerous and premature.

Question (Dr. Wolf, from audience): An implicit fact revealed at this meeting is the extreme complexity in setting-up dosage forms of reproducible bioavailability. What implication does this have on the future of small drug houses selling generic drugs and the large companies who spend the money in developing the original formulation of the drug? What is the impact on the generic drug situation?

Response (Dr. Simmons): This merely emphasizes the importance of bioavailability; it is a good reason for having a bioavailability requirement. The data would demonstrate that. In fact, it shows that one has solved the problem of drug formulation and not merely produced the same chemical entity.

Comment (from audience): The reason that non-generic drugs are not cheap is that it takes money and effort to develop the drug. It should be recognized that if a generic drug house will undertake to obtain the proper bioavailability data, it will be competitive with trademark drug houses. Thus, the problem dissolves itself away – the more you enforce requirements that a drug be good, the less likely it is that it will be cheap. Thus, drug houses should not only come up to standards but develop new standards of excellence.

Question (audience): Since this meeting has shown that the formulation characteristics of a drug are as important as the chemical characteristics, is not the secrecy of the former inopportune? Let us consider making formulation characteristics public.

Response (Dr. Macek): This is exactly our position. The definition of the composition and the process for manufacture of a drug product are a means of standardization. We should define both chemical and *in vivo* characteristics.

Comment (Dr. Weiner): This is a very important issue. However, at a professional meeting it suffices to identify the chemical structure but not the method of synthesis – usually a trade secret – for the scientist to judge your product. It is also necessary to define the conditions or properties that make this product good, e.g. dissolution time, but not to reveal the details that make it good. Thus, the following analogy can be made: compound versus the method for making compound and properties of compound versus how they are attained. This could be a real conflict but it is unnecessary.

Question (audience): What will be the effect of bioavailability requirements by the regulatory agency on preclinical toxicity testing for inclusion in IND's and NDA's?

Response (Dr. Simmons): No effect. I wish to make a comment to Dr. *Wolf*'s remark. As we discover the real complexities of drugs, one wonders how much of the world's medical literature is inaccurate. How many inaccurate judgments have been made in the past since something may have been attributed to a drug that was not due to the chemical but to some other characteristic? On this basis, how many good and bad drugs have entered and left the market?

Question (audience): If *in vitro* results do not match *in vivo* testing, do you see bioavailability tests being used for shelf-life testing and checking?

Comment (Dr. Leeson, audience): One must confront each individual problem. For example, a change in dissolution characteristics may or may not reflect bioavailability of the drug. Raising the questions leads to regulation – like retest every 2 months. You can see how this would be impractical.

Comment (Dr. Bergen): Purpose of the conference has been to lay the groundwork for routine standards, from the standpoint of the official compendia, in governing the uniformity of drug products with respect to bioavailability. It is clear that this is immensely complex and each drug product is a different problem. I do not see too much difficulty in orienting research efforts in bioavailability or the need for bioavailability data prior to marketing a new product. The question that remains is what are the guide lines going to be for evaluation on a lot to lot basis? In some cases *in vitro,* in others *in vivo* until correlations can be developed. This is reminiscent of the course of development of drug assays.

Comment (Dr. Simmons): Enlightened regulations which are derived out of consultation with those knowledgeable in the field are necessary and of benefit.

Comment (Dr. Leeson, audience): The drug industry could not exist without such protection and looks upon FDA to render that protection.

Comment (Dr. Macek): I am not sure that we are in a position or should even attempt to define standards for all drugs. We should take one step at a time. If we can succeed in developing a reference method for several drugs where a problem exists, we will have made progress. And that is the important thing.

Closing Remarks

A. Gilman

Department of Pharmacology, Albert Einstein College of Medicine, Bronx, N.Y.

At this hour, any closing remarks should be very short indeed and I promise that they will be.

In my mind, bioavailability cannot be separated from drug efficacy and safety. This problem has long been appreciated by the DRB, especially as it related to the Drug Efficacy Study.

Shortly after the inception of the review in 1966, a conference was held on 'Bioavailability' and as a result, the following statement was appended to all reports submitted to FDA.

> 'Drugs of identical chemical composition (so-called generic drugs) formulated and marketed by numerous individual firms under generic or trademarked names have been evaluated for efficacy as a group without consideration of "therapeutic equivalence". In the event that no evidence for pharmacological availability or therapeutic efficacy in man can be presented for any of the indications claimed for the use of any of the drugs in the attached listing, their classifications of effectiveness may need to be modified if regulations of the FDA require such proof.'

It is indeed gratifying that this subject is receiving the attention it deserves as exemplified by the large attendance at this conference and the scientific excellence of the papers and panel discussions. At this time I wish to express the appreciation of the DRB for the efforts of the USP and to extend our thanks to the various co-sponsors. The efforts of Dr. *Macek* in organizing the program have been richly rewarded.

Finally, it is evident that any group of consumers that supports legislation for obligatory generic prescribing of the type that denies the physician the opportunity to indicate the source of the generic drug, has no concept of the risk/benefit ratio involved. Every person in this room should make every effort to inform those involved in such legislation of its dangers and prematurity.